THINK Yourself® HEALTHY

27 SIMPLE, PRACTICAL APPLICATIONS FOR A VIBRANT LIFE

by
Nathalie Plamondon-Thomas

A companion book to the THINK Yourself® book series

THINK Yourself® HEALTHY Copyright© 2018
by Nathalie Plamondon-Thomas.

All rights reserved. No part of this book may be used or reproduced in any manner whatsoever without written permission except in the case of brief quotations in critical articles or reviews.

Disclaimer: The information in this book is for entertainment purposes only and does not constitute health advice in any way. Readers should consult with their own medical professionals before embarking on any health or mindset training.

Published by THINK Yourself® PUBLISHING. www.thinkyourself.com

The author of this book can be reached as follows:

Nathalie Plamondon-Thomas: www.thinkyourself.com

ISBN: 978-1-7753653-3-4

First Edition: June 2018

FOREWORD

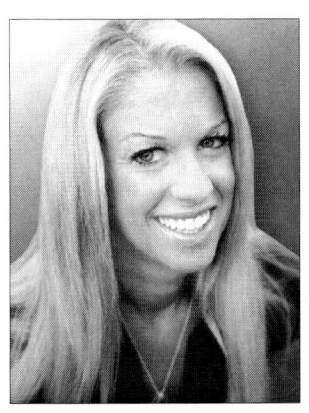

August 1992. I had just moved out of my parents' house to live in my own apartment, to go to a high-school in a different city. That was when I discovered Costco. I had no idea that you could buy full boxes of chocolate bars. Sweet! I had a couple every day during my college years.

Ten years later: I was part-owner in a printing business. We had over fifty employees. More than once a week, I would stop on my way to work and buy three or four dozen doughnuts for the staff. I would eat two or three as they were lying on the passenger seat, on my way to work, for breakfast.

December 2015. I am standing in my kitchen at 7:00 a.m., eating the remaining three portions of dessert from the night before. Suddenly, I hear a noise. Somebody is up. I quickly put what is left back and wash the spoon to make the 'evidence' disappear.

Yes, true stories. I have been there. It happens to me too. I know exactly how you feel. Me too! It is not that I don't like sweets or bad stuff. It is not that I never go there or want to. We are all in this together. Over the years and through my own personal journey, I have developed some strategies that I use for when that happens. And I will teach you the tricks I use when my devils seem to speak louder than I would like them to.

I write books on neuroscience and brain programming. I love that stuff.

A lot of readers who have read my No.1 best seller THINK Yourself® THIN tell me how much the system I shared in the book has completely changed their lives. Now that they know how to set up their brain to be on board with their health goals, they have the foundational layers to be ready to implement new skills into their lives.

Used with the full THINK Yourself® system in mind, these 27 simple and practical habits can easily find space in your life.

These tips are mine. They are what I precisely set up in my environment, what I do, what I'm good at, what I believe, who I am and why I am doing this. I am sharing this with you in a very humble way as a response to all the emails I get from people who want to know what my 'secrets' are.

Enjoy.

Nathalie

"THINK Yourself ® HEALTHY is a refreshingly efficient read about health and how to achieve it without feeling overwhelmed. A healthier you is within your grasp. I love the read."

- Tosca Reno, New York Times Best Selling Author
and Founder of the Eat Clean® Revolution.

TABLE OF CONTENTS

FOREWORD v

QUIZ ix

THE NEUROLOGICAL LEVELS 1

Part 1: BEING HEALTHY COMES FROM WITHIN 3
    The logical mind 6
    The unconscious mind 7
    Relax and ask your unconscious mind 8
    Your personal assistant 9
    The chef knows how to cook 11

Part 2: ENVIRONMENT 13
    TIP #1: Set up your environment 14
    TIP #2: Exercise with others – Surround yourself with people who exercise 18
    TIP #3: Prepare your clothes in advance to work out 20
    TIP #4: Don't have it at home 22

Part 3: BEHAVIOURS 25
    TIP #5: Plan your snacks 26
    TIP #6: Make sure you are fed 29
    TIP #7: Cheat. Sometimes 34
    TIP #8: Keep Walking 36
    TIP #9: Eat before you go for dinner or grocery shopping 38
    TIP #10: Do it. Don't think about it 39

Part 4: SKILLS 43
    TIP #11: Choose your food wisely 44
    TIP #12: Stop the pop 47

TIP #13: Have your exercise planned and stick with it...
Or improvise 49

TIP #14: Skills: Know what to eat before and after you train 60

Part 5: BELIEFS AND VALUES 65

TIP #15: Catch what you say & think 67

TIP #16: You don't need to feel full.. 70

TIP #17: Recognize when it's just a scratch 74

TIP #18: Get permanent with it 76

TIP #19: Have healthy things to make you feel great................ 77

TIP #20: Be left wanting it before the first bite......................... 83

Part 6: IDENTITY 85

TIP #21: Stop saying: "I AM FAT"... 86

TIP #22: Love yourself more than the food 88

TIP #23: Be allergic 90

Part 7: LIFE PURPOSE (The Big Why) 93

TIP #24: Know why you want to be healthy............................... 94

TIP #25: Think about the future, how long you want to live 95

TIP #26: Teach others, be the leader of a group,
have people who look up to you 97

TIP #27: Eat organic for the environment.................................. 99

SOME FINAL TIPS 102

MY MEALS 103

My breakfast 103

My lunch 105

Other Lunch ideas 105

My snacks 105

My dinner.. 106

Desserts 107

ABOUT THE AUTHOR.. 109

INTRODUCTION

Here are a series of questions to open your mind. I have designed the statements to be incomplete on purpose. Taken out of context, the sentences could be true or false. Go ahead, fill in the quiz, and compare your answers with mine as you make your way through the upcoming chapters of the book. Let's find out where your mind went when you read the questions. It may be very different from where I had intended to take you.

	Statement	TRUE	FALSE
1	The more food in your fridge, the healthier you will be.		
2	You have more chances to exercise when you feel that you have to.		
3	Exercising is all about the outfit.		
4	Far from the eyes, far from the mouth.		
5	You should always think about food.		
6	You should eat something after a big dinner when you feel really full.		
7	Cheating may be a good thing.		
8	Walking can make you lose weight.		
9	Eat before a meal to spoil it.		
10	Reflecting and thinking about something will help you actually do it.		
11	Always look for calorie count on a packaged food.		
12	Diet soda is better than regular.		
13	Exercising for less than thirty minutes is not worth it.		
14	You should not eat before a workout.		
15	Affirmations don't work.		
16	You need your food to be satisfying.		
17	When you make a terrible choice, nutrition-wise, you should keep going as though your day is a write-off anyways. You will start fresh the following day.		
18	When you lose weight, you always gain it back.		
19	Food makes us feel good.		
20	Feeling that we want to eat unhealthy stuff is wrong.		
21	If saying that we are overweight makes us overweight, then saying that we are thin will make us thin.		
22	You have to love healthy food.		
23	Lying is a good thing.		
24	Focus on what to do to be healthy.		
25	Thinking about the present will help you get to your ideal weight.		
26	You should think of what other people would think about you.		
27	Being healthy will help future generations.		

THE NEUROLOGICAL LEVELS

A person's self can be represented in six specific layers. Author Robert Dilts, who has been one of the fore thinkers of Neuro-Linguistic Programming (NLP) since its creation in 1975, identified them as the "six neurological levels". When wanting to reach a goal, it is imperative for you to address each level to reprogram your brain correctly and succeed. Making sure that your brain, the most complex and powerful structure in the universe, is on board, will fast track your success.

I have chosen to present the tips of this book to be used along with each neurological level: Environment, Behaviour, Skills, Beliefs and Values, Identity, and Life Purpose. They are the basis of the D.N.A. System that I use in all my other books. Feel free to pick up any book from the THINK Yourself® series to find out more about the whole system. In this book, I will use the six neurological levels to guide you through setting up your mindset in a way that will give you results.

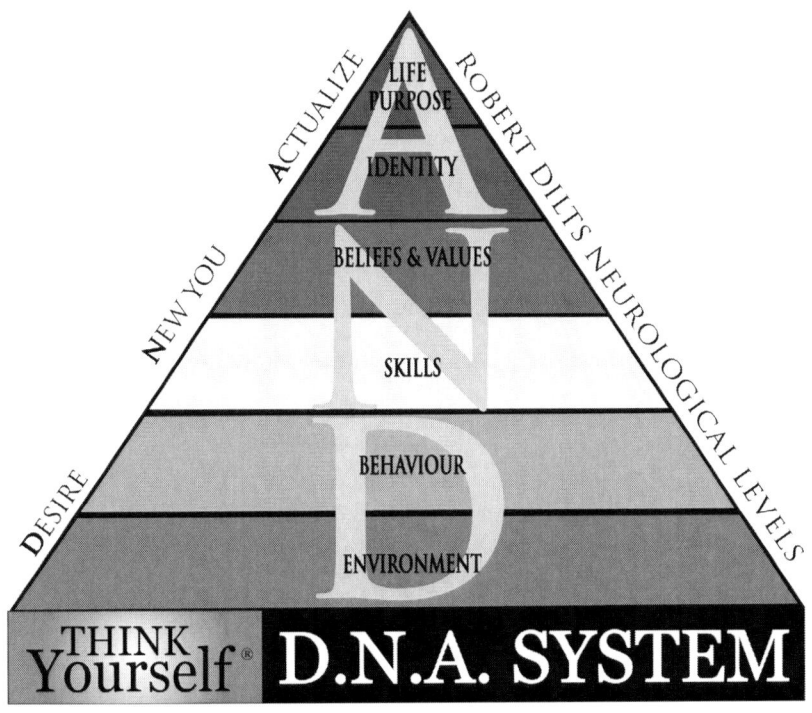

PART 1:
BEING HEALTHY COMES FROM WITHIN

Have you ever had a friend or a family member who shared with you that they had just come up with a fantastic idea? You looked at them, stupefied, wanting to shake them and say: "Dude, I have been telling this to you for two months! All of a sudden, YOU just got this idea?"

Your brain is the most complex structure in the universe. Asleep or awake, it controls every moment, every movement and every thought of your life. It records what you hear, it distorts, generalizes and deletes information to create your model of reality. Somehow, we are all the same. We like to make sense of things ourselves, and we don't listen to advice. We only act on them when we can generate the light bulb ourselves in our brain. So just like we can take a horse to water but cannot make him drink, all the tips in the world will be useless unless you decide to do something with them.

With this premise, I should not bother writing a book of tips, because as I just said, we don't like to be told what to do.

So, instead of just laying down the suggestions in no particular order, I will quickly introduce you to the astonishing powers of your brain. You are awesome, and I can't wait for you to discover it. Then I will lay out the practical tips in a specific way which will help you program each layer of your brain so that you happen to generate the idea of doing it yourself. I will show you some different ways to follow the system that I've developed, with the aim to somehow 'make the horse drink'.

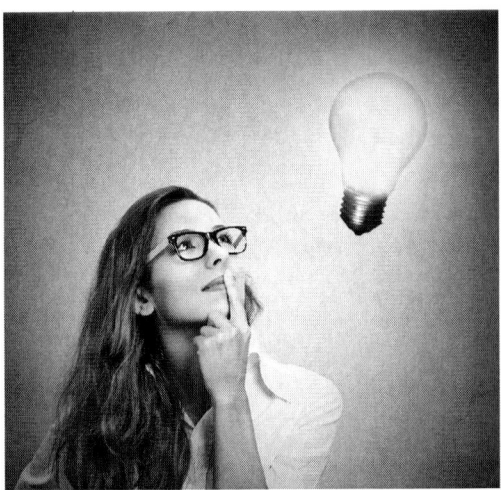

THE LOGICAL MIND

We use our logical mind on the surface in our day-to-day. Your logical mind is the voice you hear in your head all the time. The one you use to make decisions. We give our logical mind lots of responsibilities and place lots of hope on the extent of its power. The logical mind can process an average of five to nine pieces of information at the same time. While you are reading this book, you are likely also able to notice an average of seven other things.

Have you ever noticed when you are driving to a new address, as you come closer and start looking at the civic numbers on doors, you need to lower the volume of the radio in your car? Somehow, your 'five to nine' pieces of information juggled by your logical mind get filled up very quickly. As you are driving, with the foot on the brake/accelerator, noticing the red light ahead, the child about to cross the street and the weird guy in the car next to yours, somehow, doing all of this at the same time puts 'the music' into the one-too-many category, as you are adding the act of 'looking at the numbers on the houses' to all the other actions of that moment.

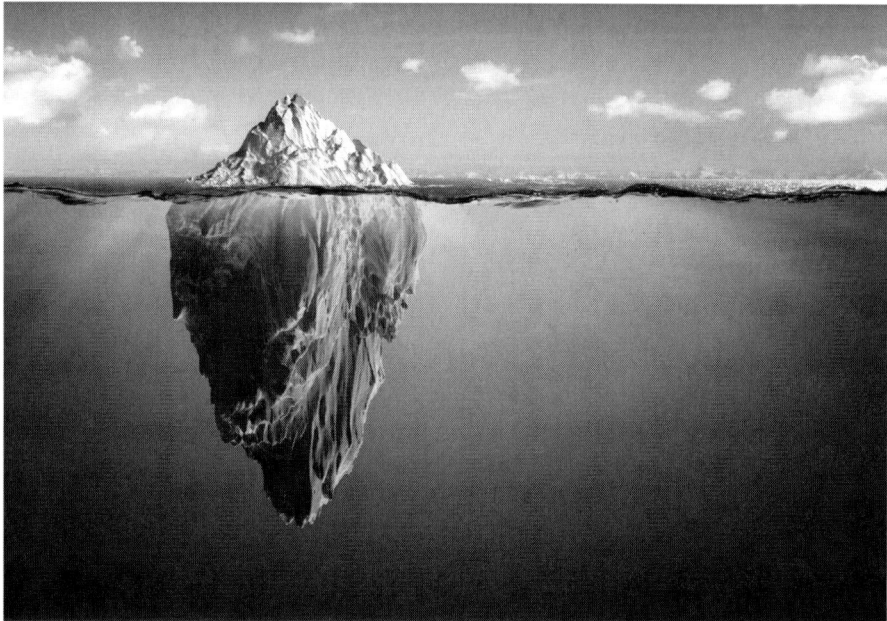

In light of this fact, knowing that we are restricted to handling only a few things at once, we may be tempted to dismiss the power of our mind. However, the logical mind is just the tip of the iceberg.

According to the research of Dr. Raj Rahunathan Ph.D., we generate between 12,000 and 50,000 thoughts per day. Unfortunately, up to 70% of these thoughts are negative. We wonder what is wrong with us? Why is everybody else successful except us? We tell ourselves we are probably not good enough. We think everyone is better and knows more than us. Sadly.

> *"Who would want to be your friend*
> *if you talked to them*
> *the same way you talk to yourself?"*
> - Unknown

Our logic might not be that great after all, right? The good news is that the voices inside your head can be reprogrammed when you discover and start connecting with the second part of your mind.

THE UNCONSCIOUS MIND

While the logical mind is busy talking down to you, the unconscious mind is busy working and understanding everything, down in the deep structure of your Self. The unconscious mind can handle over two million pieces of information every second, (while our little logical mind was only able to manage seven, on average).

Everything you have seen, done, thought, heard and felt is organized in your deeper structure waiting for your recall. Your unconscious mind considers everything. It reads all the signs and advertising while you drive to work. It hears every conversation around you, whether you are paying attention or not. It feels all the non-verbal signs that others are communicating with you without their knowledge. It captures all the "behind the scenes" detail that the logical mind misses. It takes all the info, it deletes, distorts and filters everything to create your model of reality.

Your unconscious mind has so much information for you. You have everything you need inside yourself. You got this. The problem is that people are not trained to think with their unconscious mind.

RELAX AND ASK YOUR UNCONSCIOUS MIND

Clients and friends often ask me for advice, or they want my opinion on something. The on-going response is always: "It doesn't matter what I think. I trust you know exactly what to do, you are very smart and resourceful, and you will figure it out."

It doesn't matter what I think. I was not there. I don't know all the details about this. I don't have their background, their experiences nor their values. They have to ask the only person who was there all their life; who noticed everything; who heard every conversation and even picked up on all of the non-verbal information not picked up by anyone else. They have to ask their unconscious mind. It knows exactly what to do.

The best moment to do so is at night before you go to sleep. Next time you need advice about something, before you get into bed at night, intentionally ask your unconscious mind to recall every piece of information you have on the subject and to give you a clear vision the next morning. It is essential to ask your unconscious mind to do this while you are profoundly asleep. (Otherwise, it could keep you up all night). You must specify that while your logical mind is recharging and getting long hours of rejuvenating sleep, you want your unconscious mind to work in the background, so it can give you answers in the morning.

I often use this technique when I have a deadline to write an article or a specific task. I ask my unconscious mind to write it overnight so that when I wake up the morning after, the words come quickly and effortlessly to me. I even use my unconscious mind to pack before a trip. It knows every single piece of clothing I own, it knows which ones I prefer, which ones are the most comfortable and appropriate for the trip that is ahead of me. Usually, the morning after asking my unconscious mind to make a list for me, I only need 15 minutes, and my suitcase is closed!

When you send your unconscious mind on a mission, it keeps working for you in the background as you continue to live your life. It makes sure that things happen well for you. You can use your unconscious mind like you would use a personal assistant.

YOUR PERSONAL ASSISTANT

PLACE YOUR ORDER

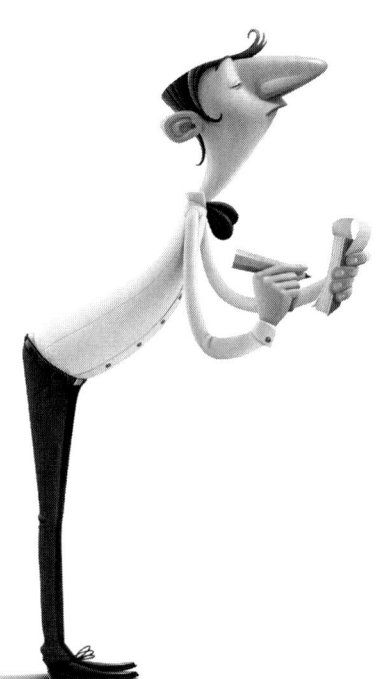

Your personal assistant inside your head takes notes and makes sure that everything that you say or think gets done. It's like having a waiter in your head, standing with a notepad and running to the kitchen to place your order.

Whatever you think or say will get cooked by the chef and brought back to you exactly how you ordered it. You have to be careful when you think and when you talk. Your personal assistant is always listening.

If you wake up in the morning and look at yourself in the mirror and say: "Oh my! I look horrible! I look so old and tired! I am so overweight," then you continue with your day saying to yourself that you feel so stupid, or inadequate, or you don't want to be stressed, and you hate rushing everywhere.

You let the voice inside your head tell you that you are a failure and a fraud, and you even tell yourself not to forget something (maybe a folder you are supposed to bring to the office). All your brain can hear is: Horrible, Old, Tired, Overweight, Stupid, Inadequate, Stress, Rush, Failure, Fraud, Forget the folder, etc.

Close your eyes for a second and do NOT visualize Mickey Mouse wearing a yellow tuxedo standing on top of an elephant. Did you see him? Of course, you did! Even if you read: "Do NOT visualize Mickey Mouse...." Your brain doesn't process negation. You have to be careful! People sit in my office all the time telling me they don't want to be stressed anymore, they don't want to be fat, they don't want to be impatient with their kids and they don't want to be rushing all the time!

It is like they are telling their contractor that they want them to paint their kitchen 'not' blue. What do you want instead? Use your brain wisely, think and say what you want, not what you don't want!

Have you heard people say: "I am terrible with names." Who decided that you were terrible with names? Who made the call? As you say that, you place an order to forget their name.

Some people say: "I am a morning person" or "I am a night owl." They conditioned themselves to be that way, and they believe it. If I need to stay up late, then I am an evening person, and if I need to get up early, then I tell myself that I am a morning person. I can be both. Whatever serves me. If a belief is not serving you, change it!

THE CHEF KNOWS HOW TO COOK

Sometimes, we undervalue our worth. We feel that we have to restrain our demands to what we know. We don't allow ourselves to dream too high because we don't know precisely how to get there.

Take the example of the waiter awaiting your order at the restaurant. When you order something from the waiter, you don't necessarily need to know how to cook the dish you have ordered. You just place your order. The chef put it on the menu, so that means that the chef knows how to cook it. The chef is your unconscious mind. She knows exactly how to make it happen. If you were able to dream it, it means that your chef knows how to cook it. You would not have been able to imagine it if you did not have what it takes to realize it.

All you have to do is to place your order with the waiter. The waiter will run to the kitchen, and the chef will gather all the ingredients to create your dish. The logical mind is not necessary for this.

When you are clear about what you want and what you expect from your unconscious mind, it starts working for you in the background while you continue to live your life. It guides you into being at the right place at the right time. It whispers answers into your ears when you are about to learn something that will generate results towards your goal. It makes you feel like doing something right. It makes you feel like exercising and eating healthy food. Trust that you have everything you need inside. You got this. Place your order!

PART 2:

You now know how the brain works. I will introduce the foundational layers of the brain, one by one, and revisit the questions from the quiz as I introduce each tip to you. Each of them belongs to one neurological level. Let's start with the tips that source in our environment.

ENVIRONMENT

Our Environment is where we live, have fun, work, and also our surroundings. It is the places we go and the people with whom we interact. People often try to identify themselves by the type of car they drive, the neighbourhood in which they live, the kind of office they have, the brand of clothes they wear. None of these represents who we are on the inside. It is just part of our environment. Becoming identified with our environment can be very positive if the environment healthily supports us. Here are a few tips that belong to your environment level.

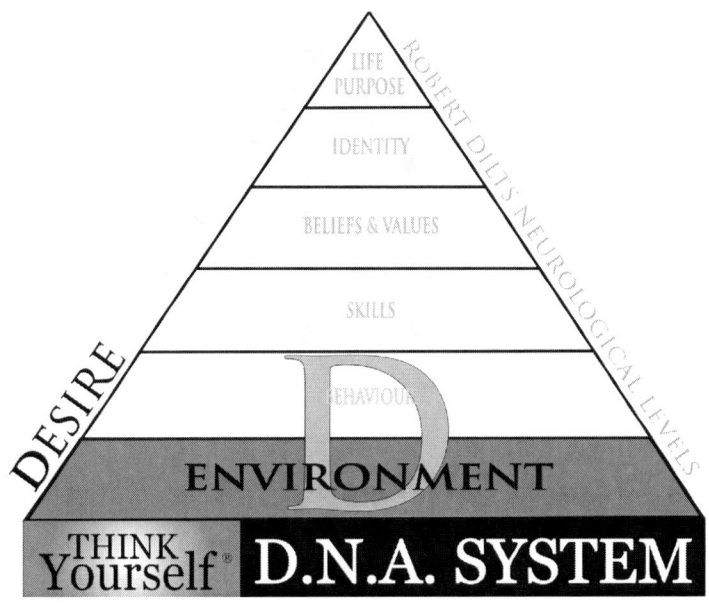

TIP #1:
SET UP YOUR ENVIRONMENT

1 The more food in your fridge, the healthier you will be.	**True** In this section of the book, you will learn about how setting up your fridge with healthy food will allow you to quickly have access to what you want to eat, instead of grabbing fast food or other unhealthy options.

Set up your environment so that everything is ready to go. The best way to stick to a plan is to have one. Decide in advance what you will be eating and prepare it ahead of time so that it is there in your environment, ready to go. There is nothing worse than opening the fridge when you are starving and grabbing the first thing that you can put your hand on, good or bad.

First, it is best if you don't have 'bad' stuff in your fridge altogether (see tip number four: Don't have it at home). Now even if we have relatively healthy food in our fridge, when we are hungry or are pressed for time, we most likely will reach for something quick and easy. If I had to start boiling quinoa and hard-boiled eggs every time I am ready to make my lunch salad, I would most likely never eat salads at all. Too much work!

I've made a habit of doing my food prep for the week on Sundays. It allows me to make sure that the salad making process is simple and appealing. Nothing exciting about a bowl of spinach with a slice of tomato. I make my salad healthy and copious at the same time. You can see the last chapter of this book where I tell you the full list of what goes in my salad. The trick is to identify your favourite foods and make sure you always have them handy and ready to be mixed. The salad making process becomes a bare five minutes' deal which increases the chances of your eating it.

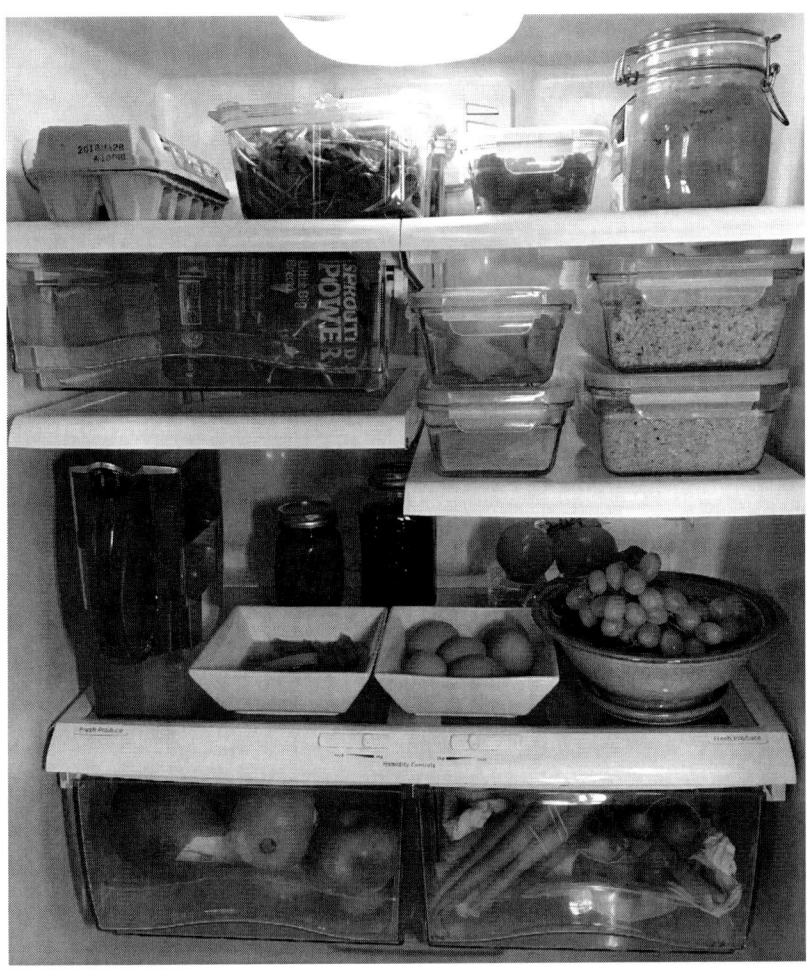

Here are a few of the foods I prepare during my Sunday routine, which takes between thirty minutes and an hour depending on the week, as I do everything at once. My process requires a little bit of multi-tasking but it is so worth it in the end.

Quinoa: I always boil 200g (1 cup) of quinoa, which takes 18 minutes. I choose either white or red quinoa which contain 8 grams of protein per cup. As I choose not to eat meat, I need some sources of protein to ensure I get the amino acids I need to keep me healthy. Quinoa also offers me a feeling of fullness, as it is one of the rare starches I eat. It also soaks up the dressing and tastes fabulous.

Eggs: I start my eggs and my quinoa at the same time. I put 7 or 8 eggs in a pot with water and use the same 18-minute timer. It takes about 8 minutes for the egg water to boil and 10 additional minutes for them to cook. When the quinoa timer rings, I take the eggs off the stove and rinse them with cold water and place them in an open bowl in the fridge, ready to grab to put in my salad or eat as a snack. Mother nature has made a perfect combo when creating eggs. Did you know that to better absorb protein, you need to also eat healthy fat at the same time? The amount of fat in the egg yolk is the perfect amount required to absorb the amount of protein present in the egg white. When people ask me what I think about using egg whites only to make an omelette, my response is always: unless your doctor told you that you had a problem with cholesterol, the egg yolk is fabulous for you. Now if your doctor said you that you had a cholesterol problem, many other things are a lot worse than an egg yolk. Remove all animal products from your diet before removing the egg yolk and once it is all out of your system, test again and more likely your doctor will be pleased with your results. I do limit my egg consumption to 7 or 8 per week.

Steel-cut oats: While the other things are cooking, I place 200g of steel-cut oats mixed with hemp hearts and sprouted chia, with 800g of water (4 times more), in a pot on the third burner of the stove. Steel-cut oats take longer to cook, and I would most likely stick to the instant stuff if I had to go through it every morning. I boil it a little longer than the quinoa. When the quinoa and the eggs are cooked, I put the eggs away, then put the quinoa in a glass container in the fridge, and then I address the steel-cut oats which have taken an extra few minutes on the heat. Because I added very-absorbent chia to the oats, and because the soaking process continues for a long time even after they are removed from the stove, I add a few hundred grams of water as I know it will continue to thicken as it cools. I leave the oats in the pot in the fridge overnight, and I store it in a glass container the following day once it has absorbed the extra water. In the morning, all I have to do is to grab a big dollop from the fridge and warm it up on the stove with a half banana or frozen fruit.

Frozen fruit: When in season, we purchase fresh fruit from local farmers: between 15 kg and 30 kg of mix-and-match berries, blueberries, raspberries, and strawberries. We clean them and freeze them on cookie sheets (which keeps them from clumping together) in the freezer for a few hours before transferring them into bags that will last us all winter. We also buy pitted cherries from a farmer in Kelowna B.C. who sells them already pitted and frozen. (Yes, I find pitting cherries a bit outside my enjoyment, so I buy them already pitted).

Veggies sticks: My husband arranges veggies such as carrots, celery, cauliflower, broccoli and peppers and puts them in a bowl of water in the fridge, for us to grab easily whenever we get the munchies. If we don't have time to prepare them, I even buy the expensive veggie trays at the grocery store. In the end, it costs me a lot less than having to miss work because of being sick. Vegetables keep me healthy.

Beets: I love beets. The darker the vegetable, the more antioxidants it contains. Beets are high in immune-boosting vitamin C, fibre, and essential minerals like potassium and manganese (which is good for your bones, liver, kidneys, and pancreas). They take much longer than the rest to cook. I start them on the fourth burner of the stove at the same time as the oatmeal, eggs, and quinoa and leave them there. They give my salad a sense of joy. When I have beets in my salads, it is like I am at the restaurant. It is like a colourful celebration in my plate. I don't peel them. I place them whole in enough water to cover them, and boil them for sometimes an hour, or until they are soft when I try to slice them with a knife. I strain them and then use yellow plastic gloves to remove the peel which comes off in seconds as I rub the beet in my hands. I place them in a glass container in the fridge and have all my ingredients ready for the week! All I have to do is to buy fresh greens!

TIP #2:

EXERCISE WITH OTHERS – SURROUND YOURSELF WITH PEOPLE WHO EXERCISE

2 You have more chances to exercise when you feel that you have to.	**True** What I am about to discuss is how being accountable to other people will help you stay true to your own goals.

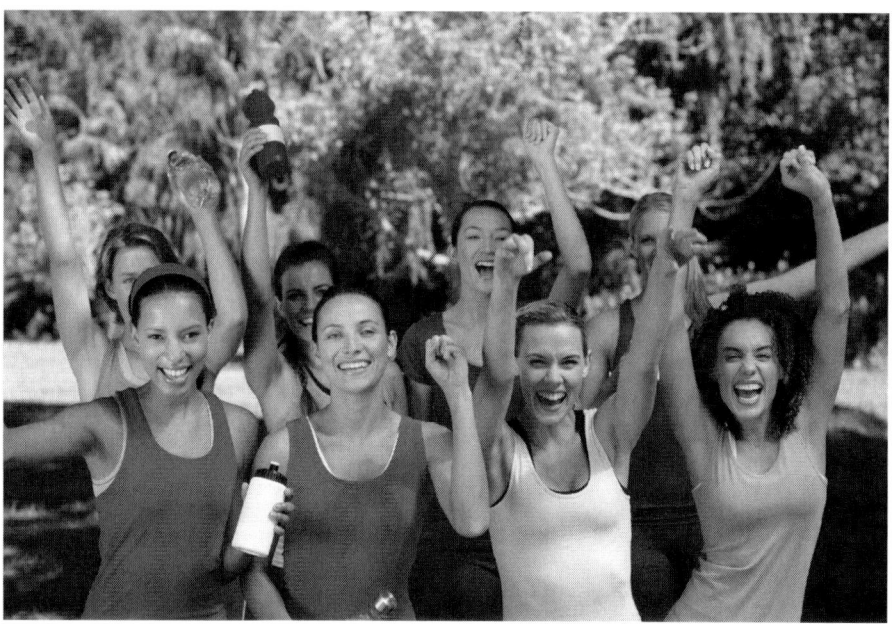

Unless it's a primary need like going to the bathroom, or an old habit engrained to happen automatically like brushing your teeth in the morning, you may not always feel like exercising. Until you do it on a regular basis and get to the point where nothing can get in the way of you and your next sweat, you may need to have a few tips to set up your environment so that it supports you in your desire to get on a healthy active lifestyle.

Hanging around people that exercise is a crucial element that will motivate you to exercise when the voice in your head is brilliantly trying to get out of it. We can be very good at making excuses. Commit to exercising with others. Set up times in advance to show up to your exercise. Run with friends. Sign up for a fitness class. If you leave it up to the end of the day and "play it by ear" as to whether or not you will feel like it, more likely, the excuses will get the best of you. Know in advance that you will exercise and do it with others.

My strategy to stay fit has been the same forever. I have been teaching fitness for over 30 years. I don't have a choice. If I don't show up, no-one is there to teach the class. I am committed. There are no nagging voices that can get the best of me. I have to show up for my participants.

I used to teach six or seven days a week, sometimes over twenty classes per week. In the past ten years, as I have changed my business significantly to do more life coaching – sitting down in my office and more writing and speaking, I am only teaching four to five classes per week, Monday to Thursday. While Saturday is my writing day and I enjoy the break from exercise, I still want to exercise on Friday and Sunday. As I don't 'have to' teach a fitness class on these days, I need to have a plan to make sure that it happens.

I had a workout buddy, and for years, we met once a week for a workout together. We would go for runs even under the worse winter conditions and talked each other through anything. We are both busy entrepreneurs who would more likely not have taken the time to go for coffee every week to catch up, but living an active lifestyle is part of our priorities. We did consider our exercise time seriously and would show up for the other no matter what. If one of us had a short-term injury, we would find a type of workout that suited the inconvenience. A sore ankle would not allow us to run so we would lift weight instead. We would make up some circuits in her garage or my gym or would go to outdoor parks and find ways to challenge each other.

We had long conversations about everything and anything as we exercised together. We would brainstorm on work or personal projects, talk about idealistic concepts and neuroscience or simply share about girl-stuff. I always looked forward to our workouts. It was my social work out of the week! So much fun!

She has now moved to Vancouver Island, and I have yet to find someone who will keep me committed to my Friday exercise. For now, on Friday, I lift weights on my own, and I have to be honest with you: the 'on my own' part is making it very easy for me to pull out. I will share with you in the next chapter my tip to make sure the Friday exercise happens.

On Sundays, I run with my husband. That makes it a sure thing. When it is me that doesn't feel like it, he talks me into it. When it is his turn to make excuses, I am the one that motivates him to tag along. Make sure to commit to something in advance and tell people that you will be there.

It is easy to find ideas. The key in this chapter is to partner up as it doubles your chances of showing up.

TIP #3:
PREPARE YOUR CLOTHES IN ADVANCE TO WORK OUT

3 Exercising is all about the outfit.	**True** Okay, I tricked you here. I meant that if you prepare your workout outfit in advance, you have more chances to show up for your exercise session.

As I mentioned earlier, with my training buddy gone, I needed to find a strategy to exercise on Fridays. I choose to exercise first thing in the morning before it's time to dive into writing, preparing a conference or seeing back-to-back clients.

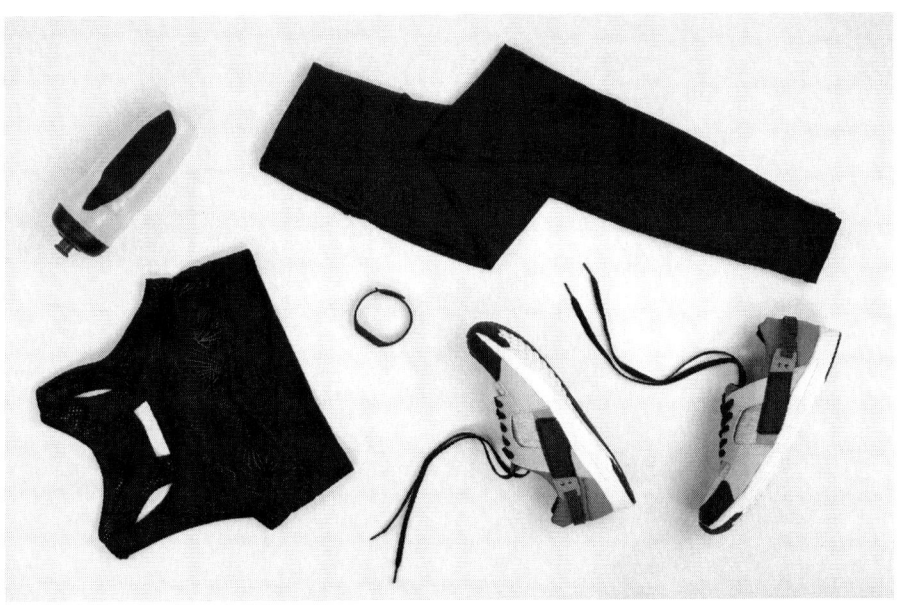

My strategy is straightforward. **I prepare my clothes in advance and leave them in the bathroom.** When the alarm goes off, as a habit which I am sure I share with a vast majority, I get up and go to the bathroom. My clothes are laying right there beside the toilet, ready to put on before I even have time to think about anything. Then I brush my teeth and start to wake up, at which time, I realize I am wearing my exercise clothes, socks, runners, etc. ready to workout. If I put the clothes anywhere else, the odds of me putting them on go down. Trust me, I have tried different areas of the bedroom.

Putting them on in the bathroom as I am still half asleep has been working for me like a magic spell. I am not noticing what I am doing, and I just do it. Once all dressed, I walk to the kitchen where I grab the shake I have prepared the night before – again, increasing my chances to go through with it – and I drink it as I walk to the gym for my short weight lifting routine.

The point of this chapter is to remember to prepare in advance. If you are planning to exercise after work, pack your bag ready to go with you in your trunk. If you happen to run into traffic, you won't use the excuse to say you did not have time to get home and grab your stuff. You can go straight to your class or workout session.

TIP #4:
DON'T HAVE IT AT HOME

4 Far from the eyes, far from the mouth.	**True** I will explain in the next chapter how avoiding having specific foods at home will increase your chance of not eating them.

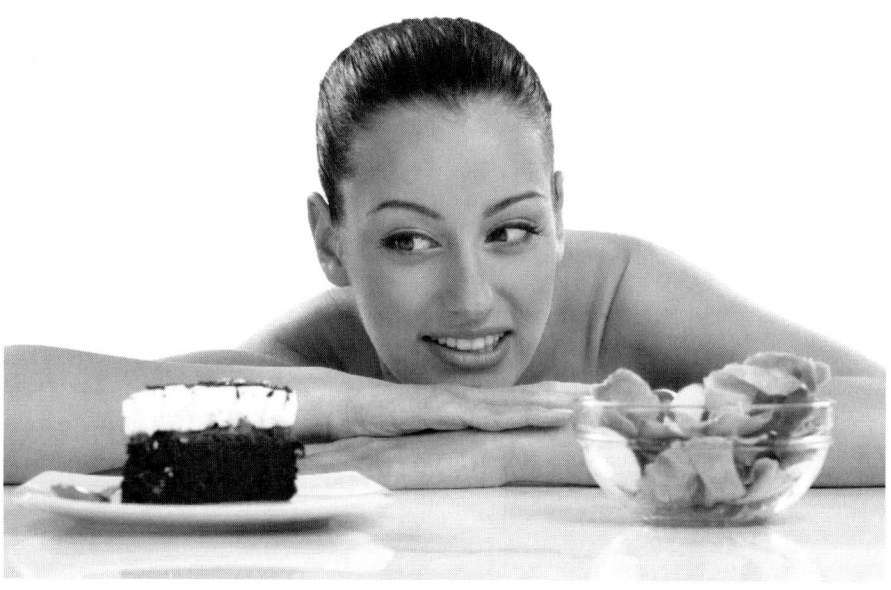

We often forget what we have in our environment. Let's pretend you choose to have a couple of rice cakes for a snack. You were honestly not even craving anything bad when you opened the cupboard to grab a light cracker and then, bam! Here it is. The box of Girl Guide cookies that your spouse bought last night is sitting right there, front and centre, torturing you. You did not even know they were there until one second ago and now that is all you can think of. They have put their spell on you. If you happen to have 'bad stuff' in your cupboards, hide it. Make it very inaccessible and especially not visible at first glance. If you remember that they are there, make it at least hard to get to.

Set up your environment so that healthy snacks are positioned strategically to wink at you every time you open the cupboard or the refrigerator. We mentioned in a previous chapter how to prepare healthy food in advance, ready to go in your fridge in order to increase your chances of eating them.

Another way to set up your environment to serve you is to make sure the bad food is out of sight, to limit its damage on your willpower. The Girl Guide cookies need to be hidden.

An even better strategy is to avoid having them in your home altogether. If it is there, of course you will be tempted. Duh! So next time you want to support a cause, just give them the money and leave them with the cookies.

Keep your fridge organized. Having a disorganized fridge that is full of old food can prevent you from eating well, because good food gets 'lost' and you may not want to deal with digging around in the messy fridge. Even if there's healthy stuff in there, you may still grab quicker, easy-to-access food.

Be very strict with your grocery shopping. Notice when your willpower seems to be at its highest, and that is when you want to choose to make your list and grocery shop. Never go when you are hungry. Go early in the morning, after breakfast or right after lunch. Only buy food that would pass the test if you were entering a clean eating contest. If you are buying food for a special occasion, buy it for that occasion only and buy just enough so that it gets entirely consumed on event day.

If you are having people over and your guests are bringing food, cheese, bread, dessert, tell them exactly how many people are expected at the party and ask that they plan for a smaller portion, a small cake, to make sure there are no leftovers. If there are some, make sure to send the guests away with them. *Do not keep compromising food in the house.*

As you will learn soon in a few chapters, if you are eating well 80 percent of the time, and allow yourself to indulge 20 percent of the time, *make sure you do so when you go out.* Keep your own house clean of unwanted temptations. Keep your car, your couch, your kitchen chairs and stools, your office chair free of any relationship with unhealthy food. The last thing you want is to anchor the memory of a piece of pie with your favourite spot on the couch in front of the television. No wonder why you would start craving pie every time you sit on that particular spot.

If you are going to be 'bad', do it somewhere other than your usual environment. It also makes sure you choose individual servings. For example, it is very rare that you will go out for dessert in a restaurant and order a whole cake, or two pieces of pie. The external pressure of having to ask the waiter for another piece will help in keeping you from eating a second serving. Interesting how we would never do this in a restaurant and somehow if there is a whole pie in the fridge, we may have two or even three portions back-to-back.

Keep your 'bad' food out of your normal environment.

PART 3:
BEHAVIOURS

Our behaviour is how we interact with family, friends and co-workers. It is what an observer may see, hear or feel when watching us engaged in a particular activity. Behaviours are the things you DO. You go to work. You brush your teeth. You eat, you walk, you drive, you exercise, you watch television, etc.

Sometimes our behaviour is consistent with the success we say we want, and other times it is not. When it is not, it is often because change needs to happen at a different level. Implementing a behaviour, like eating well or exercising, won't be useful if the problem lies at the level of 'Beliefs and Values' or 'Identity'. You will see later how these levels also need to be addressed to get the benefit of our behaviours entirely.

For now, let's learn about the ways that some specific behaviours can help with your health goals.

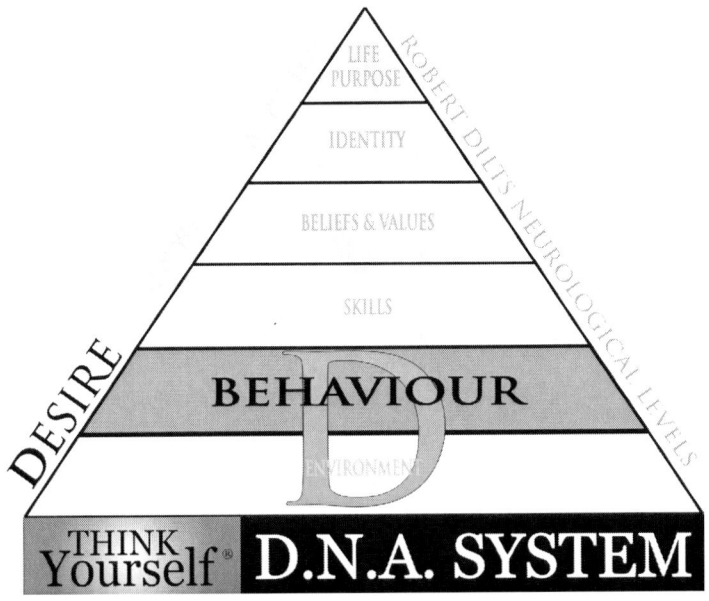

TIP #5:
PLAN YOUR SNACKS

5 You should always think about food.	**True** As mentioned, taken out of context, the statements in the quiz may be tricky. What I mean here is that you should always remember to plan your snacks and know in advance what you will eat when hunger strikes.

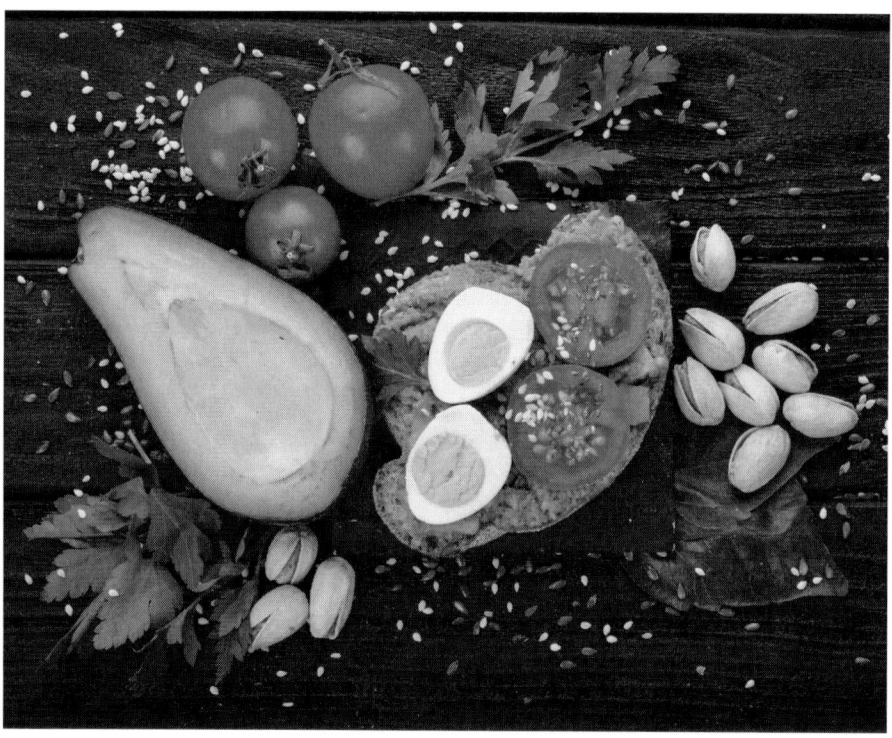

There is a lot to say about hunger. You will learn how biology works in a few chapters. While lots of our brain signals for hunger are confused with thirst signals, - yes very often, when we think we are hungry, we are simply thirsty – when we are hungry, we can devour pretty much anything, and we will grab whatever is the closest or easiest.

Prepare cut veggies in advance and leave them in an open bowl with water in the fridge on the prime spot so that it is the first thing you will see when you open the refrigerator. If you find that cutting veggies is not for you or that you attempted to buy vegetables many times and somehow forgot them in the fridge drawers until the mould and smell reminded you to throw them out, you can opt for purchasing the pre-cut-for-you veggie trays at the grocery store. Yes, they are expensive; however, they are much cheaper than any diet programs, new clothes because yours don't fit anymore, the costly impulse gift you just bought yourself to make you feel good to compensate for the fact you are unhappy with your weight, or missing work because you are sick. Investing in your health includes spending maybe a little extra on food and a lot less on other things that may be costing a lot more.

The most important thing, is getting the healthy food inside of you, and doing whatever it takes to get it there. Everything else will follow.

If you snack in the evening, plan to have the kettle ready to go, a tea bag or a portion of loose leaves in a cup waiting for you to turn on the kettle and enjoy a lovely tea instead of your calorific evening snack. If you feel like crunchy, have snap peas. If you feel like sweet, cut up an apple or a mango. Have everything handy.

If you want to make shakes in the morning, find a permanent spot on the counter so that you don't have to take the blender in and out of a cupboard every day. Make life easy for yourself.

If you buy Halloween candies more than a day in advance of handing them out, store them in the garage or somewhere you will not see them until it is time to get rid of them.

Never leave home without food and water. Water is the first thing you should think about. Very often, we confuse the thirst and hunger feelings. If you have water with you and remember to drink it on a regular basis, more likely, the food cravings will be less frequent. You will at least avoid all the ones that were caused by thirst.

Carry snacks with you. I have gotten into the habit of carrying a small bag of nuts with me in my purse. It is always there. Whenever I am leaving a meeting and am tempted to stop and grab something to eat, the nuts make me wait until I get home where food is much healthier than whatever I could have bought on my way back. I even eat nuts when I am on my way to breakfast, lunch or dinner. In many cases, functions and events start later than my usual time to be hungry, and by the time it is time to eat, I am completely starving. Eating nuts on my way there satisfies my appetite for a bit so that I can wait for the main course without overeating or without succumbing to the bread and appetizers presented to me.

Another interesting fact about nuts is they contain good fat. The fat sends a signal to your brain that tells you you're full. It takes about twenty minutes for the signal to make it to your brain. By eating a few nuts about twenty minutes before your meal; it will send a signal to your brain that you're full by the time you start eating. You'll keep your portions smaller.

How much are a few nuts? A handful. Whatever doesn't fit in your hand is too many. I count about 12 for almonds and 8 for other bigger nuts.

Apples are also my go-to when it comes to carrying food with me. I don't carry a bag of apples in my purse at all times like the nuts, but I usually just grab one from the fridge or the fruit basket on the counter when I leave home. If you place your fruit basket by where you leave your car keys, you increase your chances of grabbing a piece of fruit on your way out.

Dates. Beautiful Medjool dates are my favourite snack after a workout. I keep them in my gym bag and eat one, or two, after a workout. I use them before a workout as well, in the eventuality that I did not have time for a pre-workout shake.

TIP #6:
MAKE SURE YOU ARE FED

6 You should eat something after a big dinner when you feel really full.	**True** If you have eaten junk food that has no nutritional value, you have not been fed properly. This chapter explains how biology works.

You have learned in my first book When You're Hungry You Gotta Eat how biology works. When you understand how your body works, you will have a much easier time making healthy choices. We accuse willpower of sabotaging our dieting efforts because it's an excuse for making bad choices. **Willpower does not help overcome hunger, because hunger is a biological function.** Your brain will slow you down when you are hungry. A workout on an empty stomach feels hard because your mind is telling you to slow down and refuel. The hunger feeling is a very powerful survival instinct.

The satiety centre is an area in the hypothalamus. That's the area where your brain processes the hunger information. There are two different types of players in this area. The eating chemicals, driven by NPY, (a protein called Neuropeptide Y), and the satiety chemicals led by CART (cocaine-amphetamine-regulatory transcript). NPY decreases metabolism and increases appetite. CART stimulates the surrounding hypothalamus to increase metabolism, reduce hunger, and increase insulin to deliver energy to muscle cells rather than be stored as fat.

When you are hungry, NPY will slow you down. It will not let you use your energy because it is afraid you will run out of fuel. It slows your metabolism down. You have an empty stomach, you are starting your workout, and somehow you don't feel like it's going to be a good workout. You just can't feel the energy, and you feel weaker than usual. You hear messages in your mind like "I don't know what is going on, I'm doing the same workout as usual, but today is so much harder." You then start wanting to eat. Your brain is telling you to slow down because it's in need of energy. The light of your gas gauge is on—you need fuel. NPY increases your appetite.

The CART is the reverse. When you have enough food in your stomach, these brain chemicals send the brain a signal to increase your metabolism. The body is ordered to raise the level of energy. And your brain receives a message that now the stomach is full of energy, so it tells the body to go ahead, spend some energy, I'm good to go, I have a full tank! Then you can start running and working out with energy, or you can go back to work after a healthy lunch and start to concentrate again, see things clearly, and move with vigour. CART decreases your appetite. You need some good food in order for your brain to receive the signal that it's okay to start moving again.

LEPTIN & GHRELIN

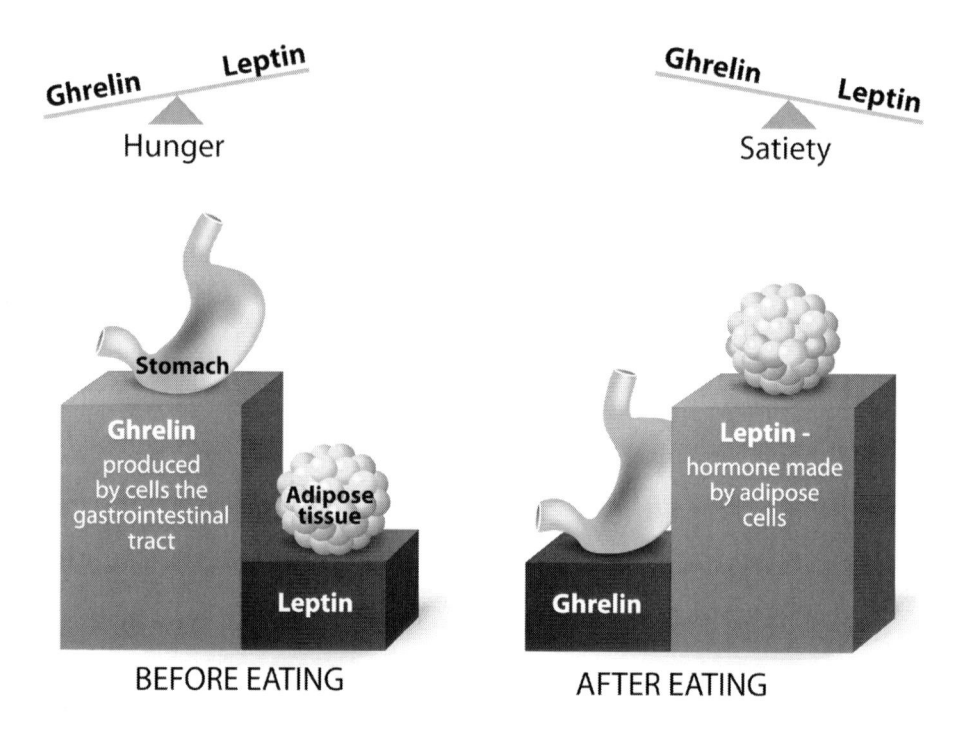

Hunger: Ghrelin / Leptin

Satiety: Ghrelin / Leptin

BEFORE EATING
- Stomach
- Ghrelin — produced by cells the gastrointestinal tract
- Adipose tissue
- Leptin

AFTER EATING
- Leptin — hormone made by adipose cells
- Ghrelin

Who is giving these signals to the brain?

The ghrelin and the leptin are both stress hormones, and they work with the NPY and the CART.

The ghrelin works hand in hand with the NPY. When you have used up your fuel, the ghrelin will transmit the signal to the NPY area of the brain. (I call it the "Gremlin" to remind myself which one is which.) The ghrelin is the little voice that tells the brain: I'm hungry. Have you ever heard that voice? As a human, your very first instinct is to survive. When you are hungry, you will listen to that ghrelin tell you every thirty minutes, then every twenty minutes, then every fifteen, ten, and then soon, if you still don't feed yourself, eating will be the sole thing on your mind.

The leptin is the satisfactory hormone. It will stimulate the CART. It will get information from your stomach and notice if it is being fueled. When it notices real food in the stomach, it will give the message to the CART area of the brain to say that it's okay to move and spend energy again.

You can read more about the anatomy of appetite in the book by Drs. Oz and Roizen called YOU: On a Diet.

IN LAYMAN'S TERMS

Here's how I can explain that to you again in my own words.

This mechanism only works with real food. Your body is smart. Your body notices what you eat. Surprise! You can't just put a chocolate bar in your mouth and hope that your body will not notice. It will.

Let's say, for example; it's lunchtime. You had breakfast before work, you may even have had a snack, an apple, a rice cake, or something similar around 10:00 a.m. and now you're ready for lunch. You have not brought your lunch with you. You go to your favourite coffee shop and get a ham and cheese sandwich. It tastes great, and you think you feel full.

But what does your body say? Your gremlin (ghrelin) is yelling, asking for food. It sees this sandwich coming in. It says great! I love ham and cheese sandwiches. What's this? Bread. Cool! Fibre and carbs are coming. But wait a minute. Your body doesn't recognise the refined and processed white bread, so it decides to just put it aside for now and stores it—on your butt, your thighs, your stomach, anywhere it can. The ghrelin keeps asking for more food.

What about the ham? That's protein, right? But, it's processed meat, and again your body doesn't recognise it. It decides to store that too. Next, we have some cheese. Great! Dairy and protein together! But it's processed cheese, and your body doesn't know what it is. What does it do with it? Stores it! Same with the mayo.

The ghrelin keeps asking for more and more food and will not shut up until you feed it. At the end of your lunch, all you've really eaten is a slice of tomato and a piece of lettuce! Vegetables. But with that, you're only good for a few minutes. It's no wonder you are hungry again in an hour. You haven't actually been fed properly.

What do you do at the end of the meal with that gremlin still yelling for food in your brain? You get an oatmeal-raisin cookie. A bit of oat may help, and a few raisins are good, but all the refined sugar will offset it, cause you to feel worse, and be stored with the rest of the junk. So, lots of garbage just added to the pile of unwanted inches covering your body. It's just stuffing yourself with "stuff" that is not real.

Now keep your attention on the next lines because we are not done here. Some of you are thinking right now that it's okay to store some garbage stuff when you work out a lot. You believe that the stuff accumulated on your bum at lunchtime will get out at 6:00 p.m. when you hit the gym.

Here is the hard truth. With no proper fuel, when you do your workout, you crash. Your workout does not fix the problems you ate.

As an example, when you are hungry yourself, do you open the refrigerator door, or the garbage bin to look for food? You want fresh, good energy, right? So, when your body needs fuel, it looks for good fuel. It won't take the fat and garbage that it did not want in the first place. It stored it once. It will not run to the trash at the first sign of hunger.

If you are not eating fuel, you are stealing it from your body. If the glycogen store is empty, your body will look for protein for fuel. It might take some energy from your muscles and bones, and then your workout makes you actually weaker than you were before. It will shrink your muscles, making you lose muscle mass, not fat. The garbage will still be there, but the muscles will be shrinking, changing your body composition.

The same phenomenon happens when you skip a meal. Some people have this very unhealthy way of losing weight: They just don't eat. They skip a few meals and then they think that they are losing weight. Truth is, they are losing muscles and bone density.

How do you get rid of your garbage? You need to contract your muscles, so they get rid of the accumulated fat. Therefore, it is essential that you feed yourself before your workout. Real food. You have to have the energy to squeeze appropriately.

A BIG DINNER, BUT NOT FED

I went out for dinner with my husband to one of our favourite Italian restaurants. We like pasta as a rare treat. Restaurants usually use white refined flour, unfortunately. That is one of the reasons why I make my own pasta because I can control what kind of flour I use. At that Italian restaurant, that day, they did not use whole flour. The meal tasted fantastic, of course, but was not healthy! We started with the warm bread dipped in extra virgin olive oil and balsamic vinegar. Yum! Then we had some pasta for our meal. And as a treat, we shared a slice of chocolate cake for dessert. Once in a while, it keeps me sane to eat unreasonable food like this.

We walked back home from the Italian restaurant absolutely stuffed. But yet, when we got home, I made myself an almond butter toast before bed. My husband looked at me and said, "Are you crazy? We just ate a huge meal!"

But the problem is that I had not been adequately fed. The bread was white bread, the pasta was white pasta, and we all know there is nothing healthy in chocolate cake. There was nothing I had in my meal that fed my body. It tasted great, and I loved it, but I had to teach a fitness class in the morning, and I knew I couldn't do it if I didn't feed my body. You have to make up for your mistakes, and that doesn't mean starving yourself because starving doesn't help. It means getting back on track and fueling your body correctly. It allows you to work out properly and get rid of the 'improper stuff'.

TIP #7:
CHEAT. SOMETIMES

7 Cheating may be a good thing.	**True** In this chapter, I explain how cheating your way to health may be the way to go for you. Going from eating fast food every day and dessert at every meal to a strict celery stick and cucumber diet may fail. Allow yourself a transition time to progress your healthy meal rate slowly.

As you read in the previous chapter, I sometimes eat 'nasty' stuff. Living a perfect life where we strictly eat clean food all the time can tint our pre-conceived notion of freedom. If we feel that we have no choice and that we are never allowing ourselves anything–although you have learned in *THINK Yourself ® THIN* how to reprogram your brain to crave healthy food and to enjoy putting healthy food in your body–we may experience feelings of restriction.

Here is how I see it. Let's say I am craving something sweet or something specific. Let's pretend I was not able to send my guests back home with their leftover dessert they brought the night before and that it is sitting in the fridge. I am tempted to have a piece of that cherry pie after dinner. All I can think of is that homemade treat that my girlfriend made with the new cherries of the season, even though I am not hungry anymore.

However, because of the presence of the cherry pie in the fridge, I feel that I 'need' something else. I grab a date. It tastes fabulous. I love dates. The feeling only lasts a few minutes as the image of the pie comes back to my mind. I then open the fridge and cut a mango. I place half in a container and eat the other half, slowly, savouring every bite. I love mangos, they can be really sweet when in season.

Of course, the image of the pie comes back. It is there, it is accessible, I can almost smell it and hear its call from the fridge. I go back to the fridge and eat the other half of the mango. Later on, of course the pie temptation comes back and now I have a bowl of cereal with half a banana. Sooner or later, I will eat the pie. In this case, if I ate it earlier at the first temptation, I would have avoided the dates, the mango, the bowl of cereal, etc. You have to recognize when it is hunger and when it is that you really want it. After all, I could have just gotten rid of it and chucked it in the garbage. I had not. It was there. Knowing myself, I revert to a previous rule when I mentioned to not have it at home altogether. That is a better strategy. Sometimes, you just want to do it and you should feel that you can.

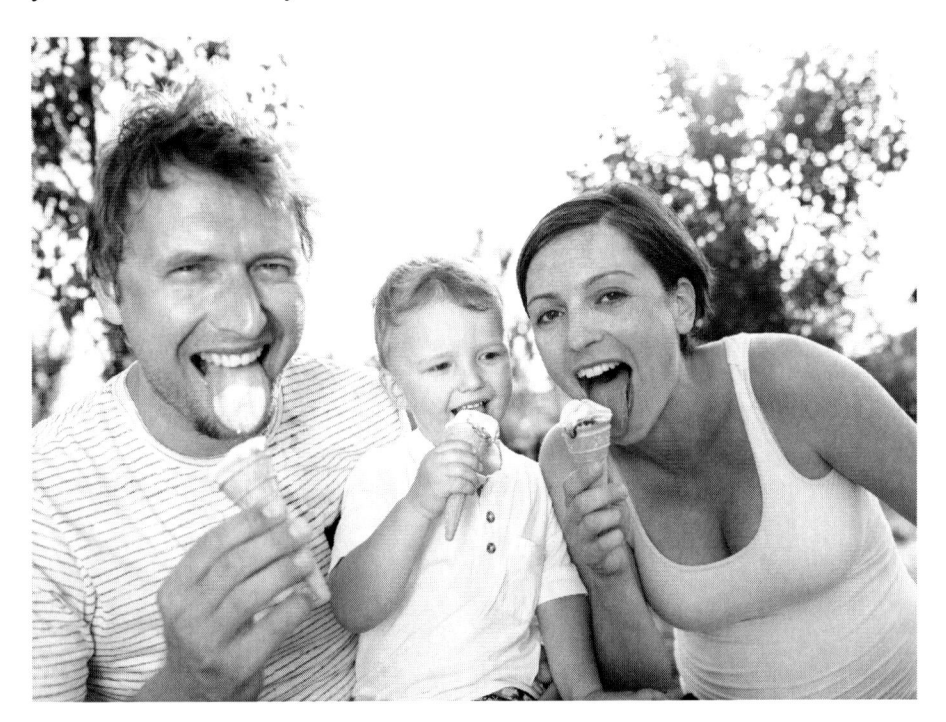

Be great eighty percent of the time. Aim for ninety. Have a small slice of birthday cake once in a while, a few fries from your friends' plate, ice cream on the beach on a hot day, etc. And when you do so, watch your language. Make sure you tell yourself that your normal is very healthy and that this moment is just an exception to your 'normal'. You will see in the chapter: "Recognize when it's just a scratch" how to correctly react when you allow yourself a few missteps.

Do one thing at a time. Living a perfect life without any 'cheating' moments can be very intense and generate lots of frustration. Depending on if you are starting your weight loss journey or if you have been eating healthy for a long time, your idea of 'cheating' may be very different from someone else's.

The 80/20 rule would imply that you eat healthy eighty percent of the meals of the week and you can let loose for the other twenty percent. If you are starting and you are at 10/90, you may want to start with aiming for eating healthy at least one day of the week. Then two, then three, etc. until you can reach the 80/20 ratio.

TIP #8: KEEP WALKING

8 Walking can make you lose weight.	**True** You more likely got this one right. However, I was not referring to the same 'walking' that you may have thought when you first read the question. Find out more in this chapter.

We saw in the environment section how surrounding yourself with healthy food will contribute to reaching your health goals.

Now here is a behaviour to increase your chances of not having bad food in your cupboards or ultimately, ending up in your stomach. There are so many temptations everywhere. Grocery stores are filled with unhealthy options and pseudo-food. Wherever we drive there are fast food drive-throughs, where calories are abundant and yet not nourishing.

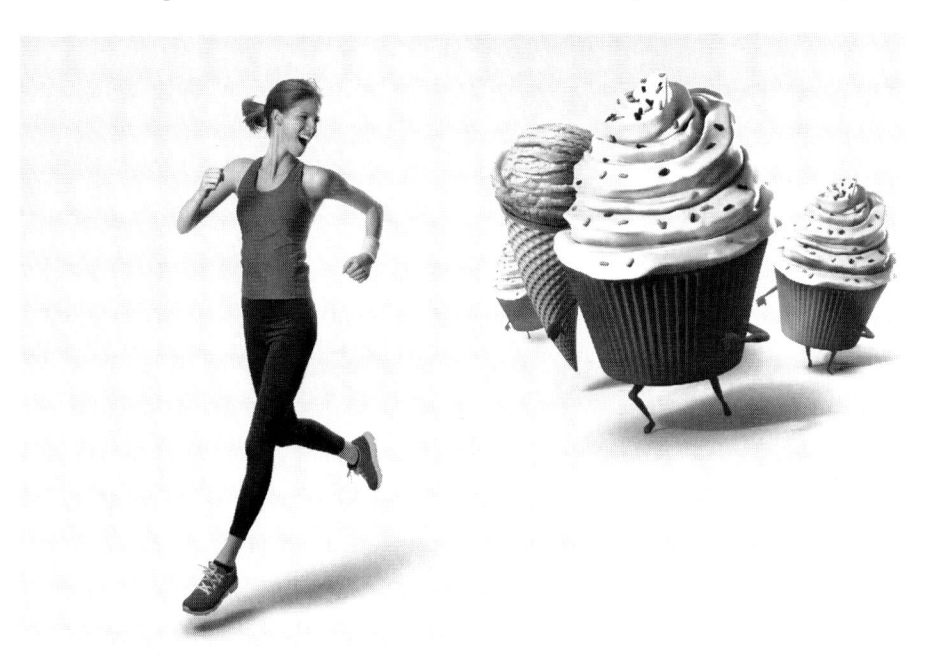

Walk away from it. When you go grocery shopping, make a list of everything you want to buy and stick to the list. Do not even enter the bakery aisle or the chips aisle. Whatever has been your downfall, up until now, will change later on as you make changes in the Beliefs section of the book. For now, repeat to yourself: "Walk away now", or "Keep walking" every time you happen to be in the presence of something you know you should not eat.

If you go to a networking event, stay away from the buffet. Choose to have a long conversation with the person standing the furthest away from the food. Chew on gum or have a mint in your mouth so that space will be occupied by something else and not as easy to stuff something in it as a result of a vulnerable moment. If you happen to walk by a plate of temptations, walk away quickly.

The same rule applies when you are contemplating sitting on the couch as you are on your way to the gym. Say it in your head: "Keep walking".

TIP #9:
EAT BEFORE YOU GO FOR DINNER OR GROCERY SHOPPING

9 Eat before a meal to spoil it.	**True** Sorry. Another trick. You will see what I mean in this chapter.

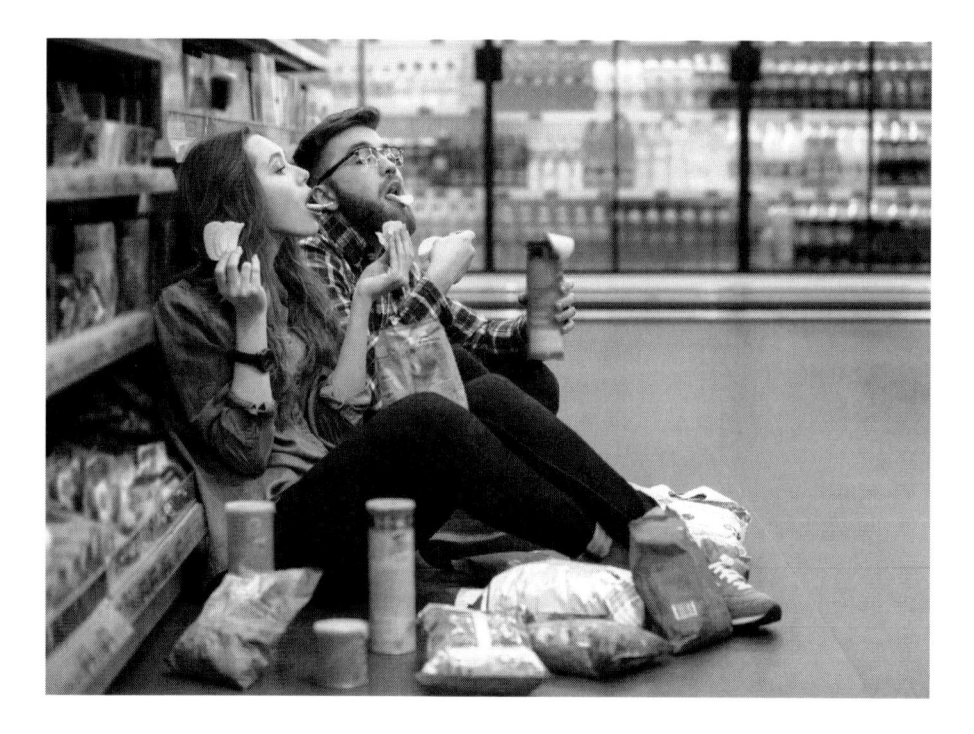

You may have heard this before. "Don't eat before the meal; you will spoil your dinner". I would like to present you with the next tip: Spoil your dinner. Yes. Do it.

Have a bowl of soup before going. Not only will you save money on an appetizer, but you will also be able to resist the bread, and your order choice will more likely be smaller or healthier than if you are entirely starving.

I know you may say: "Well, that will double the amount of food that I will eat if I eat before I go." The key is to keep it in mind when you place your order at the restaurant. Saying to everyone else: "I had a late lunch and I am not really hungry" or "I already had an early dinner", will allow you to avoid their comments on the small amount of food you are ordering.

You also have to remind yourself of it. You may think: "An appie is not enough food for me." Make sure you tell yourself too. "I ate already, so this small appetizer is perfect for me and will be plenty of food." You will see later in the upcoming chapters how to change the belief that you need a lot of food to fill you up. Have a few nuts a half hour before your meal so that you will already feel full when you start eating, and you will eat less.

Eating before you go to friend's house is also ideal, especially if you know that the place where you are going will have not-so-healthy options.

The rule also applies for running errands. Always make sure you go grocery shopping on a full stomach. There is nothing more detrimental than to shop on an empty stomach. When you are starving, you get tempted by items that may not be on the list.

TIP #10:
DO IT. DON'T THINK ABOUT IT

10 Reflecting and thinking about something will help you do it.	**False** Nope. Not in this chapter. I am referring to the fact that when we start overthinking, we find excuses to not take action. Here is what I mean.

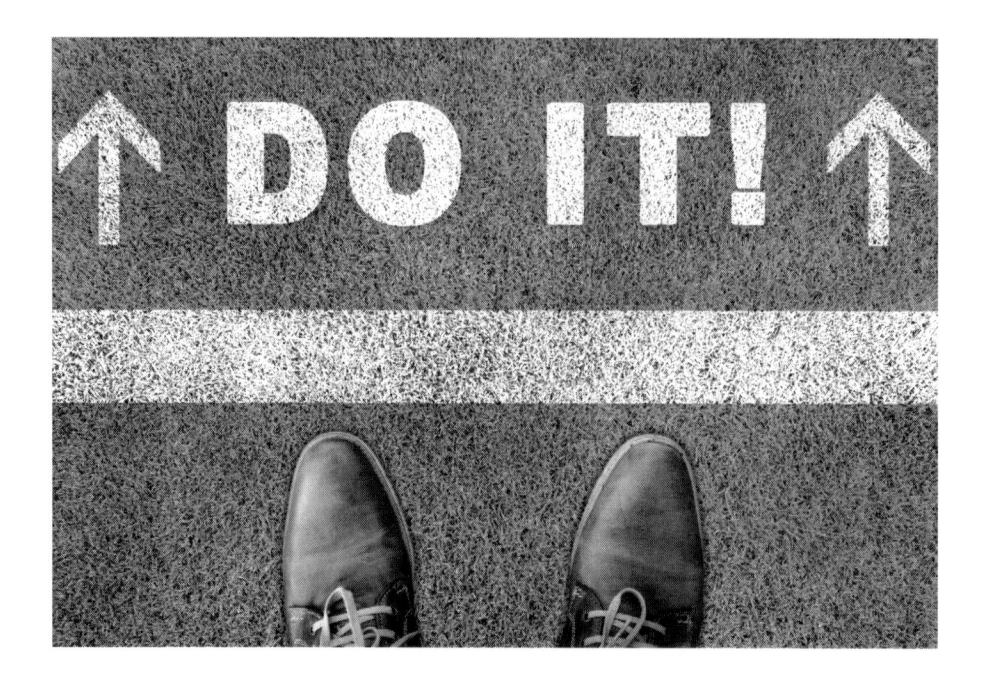

You are about to leave for the gym. As you are opening the closet to grab a jacket, you glance outside and notice it is pouring rain. Immediately, your brain starts the process. "It is miserable outside; maybe I should stay home and work out here." You put your jacket away, and you head downstairs to the small gym area set up in your basement. "I will warm up on my treadmill and then do a few weights."

If you had been at the gym, you would have had to fill up your bottle of water at the fountain, but since you are home, you can just as easily get a glass of water from your kitchen, so you head back upstairs. When you get there, you think: "We keep a pitcher of cold water in the fridge, so I will use that one." You open the refrigerator, and you see some leftovers from the night before, and you think: "I am kind of hungry, maybe I should have a little bite to eat before my workout."

You take a few minutes to wolf back some food and feel a little full, so you think that now that you ate, you will have to wait a little bit before you start your workout because you want to give your stomach a few minutes to digest. Then the devil shows up on your shoulder and whispers in your ear: "You should skip the workout altogether, you will go to the gym tomorrow…" and before you know it, you are sitting on the couch and have cancelled your exercise plans.

The first behaviour you want to adopt when it comes to making good choices for your health is to *do it*. **When you have a goal, and you know what you should be doing, just start**. It is effortless to come up with excuses when we take the time to think about it. Start. Do it. No excuses. If it rains outside, grab a raincoat and an umbrella.

Mel Robbins[1] wrote: "If you have an impulse to act on a goal, you must physically move within 5 seconds, or your brain will kill the idea. Move. Because when you physically move, your brain starts to build new habits. When you do something you're not used to doing, you are in the act of creating new habits and forgetting existing ones." Countdown in your head: "Five, four, three, two, one" then start doing what you know you should do.

---

[1] Mel Robbins, *The 5 Second Rule: Transform Your Life, Work, and Confidence With Everyday Courage*

PART 4:
SKILLS

Our skills are behaviours that we are really good at. We have innate capabilities and learned skills for dealing appropriately with an issue. We are not necessarily born with abilities. We develop them as we age with our life experiences.

When we use our skills and do what we are good at, we more likely feel in harmony with ourselves. When using our skills, we avoid that sense of wasting our talent. You have probably heard the saying: "Choose a job you love, and you will never have to work a day in your life". In this context, it makes total sense. When we are good at something, we more likely love doing it. And we love doing more of it.

What are you really good at? What are the things that are very easy for you to do without even thinking about them? What skills give you confidence and strength? What skills have you gained in the past years that support your health? What are some skills that you want to get better?

Here are some tips connected to the skills level. More than just behaviours, they are specific actions that you may choose to commit to improving.

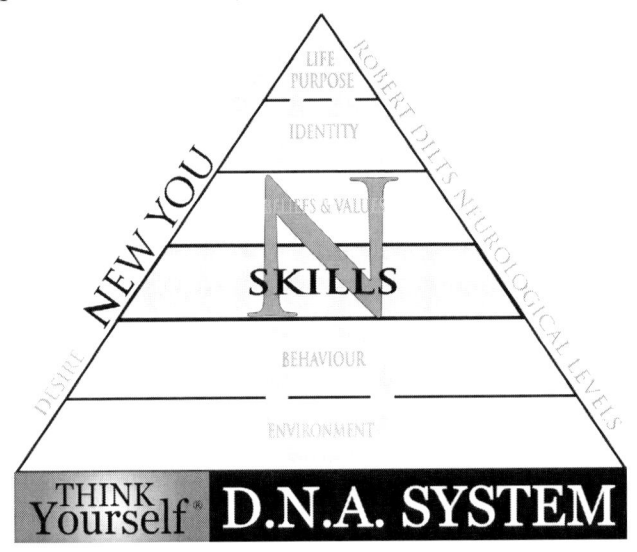

TIP #11:
CHOOSE YOUR FOOD WISELY

11 Always look for calorie count on a packaged food.	**False** Calories don't mean much. Packaged food should be avoided. But if you do have to, make sure you read the ingredients carefully.

BUY REAL FOOD

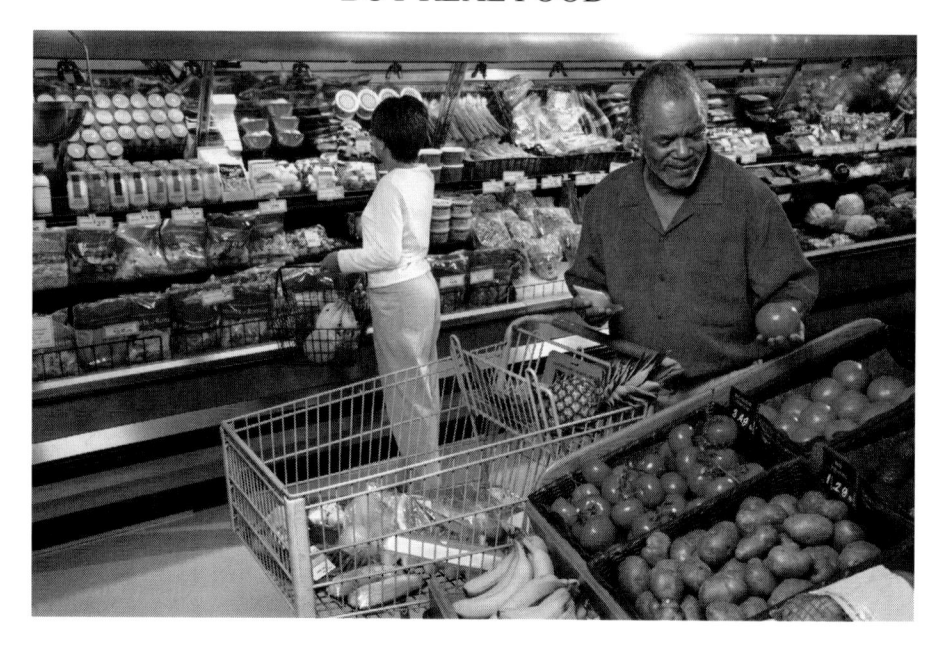

Shop around the outside edges of the supermarket. These are the produce, dairy, and meat departments. Avoid the aisles where the pre-packaged and processed foods are. These are often made up of ingredients that are not real food.

When reading the package, don't look at the number of calories or grams of fat. **Look at the entire ingredient list.** The shorter the ingredient list, the better. You should recognise the ingredients. If you don't, the chances are that it's not real food! Eat real food. Consume food that looks the same as when it was growing.

Make sure to eat real food only. Check that everything listed is pronounceable and that you know what it is.

Always make sure you read your labels. Even if someone tells you that they like a particular brand of crackers or juice, don't believe them immediately. Read it for yourself. Aim to continually increase your knowledge by reading those labels and knowing what you are eating.

STOP COUNTING CALORIES

So many calorie comparisons make me laugh. Like the one that stipulates that a salad contains as many calories as a burger and fries. It could be true. If you load the salad with a lot of healthy food, like avocado, hard-boiled egg, chickpeas, quinoa, first-cold-pressed oil, olives, even if they are healthy, they are calorific. What these nonsense comparisons don't tell you is that at least in the salad, the calories are not empty. They will feed you. Your body will know what to do with it, and your system will produce energy. Unlike when eating deep-fried potatoes.

I would much rather have a date or two, which can add up to 140 calories and which will turn my body into a fat-burning machine and provide me with energy, versus eating a 100-calorie bag of "low-cal" chips or cookies which will be deposited on my butt and will steal muscles from my body in order to get rid of it, making me weaker and will tax my digestive functions making me vulnerable to illnesses.

Understanding the load of information that is shovelled to you each day is your best way of staying healthy. Even if your doctor is telling you to eat slices of fake cheese because it's a portion of dairy, don't believe it. Check for yourself. Even if the ad on television says that the hazelnut chocolate spread contains proteins and should be given to kids, check out the remaining ingredients. It is loaded with sugar. Don't trust anyone. Read your labels!

Added sugar is in abundance in almost all pre-packaged foods. It causes cravings and addictions to foods with no nutritional value. Stay away from the '-ose' ingredients such as glucose, fructose, sucrose, dextrose, and others. Use natural sugars instead: maple syrup, honey.

ANTIOXIDANTS

We need antioxidants to fight the lactic acid that the muscles produce when working out. Antioxidants combat free radicals released during exercise that can compromise your body's natural defence. Also, avoid overtraining. Think of colourful foods with high levels of antioxidants like squash, tomatoes, carrots, pomegranates, blueberries, blackberries, olive oil, sweet potatoes, walnuts, kidney beans, broccoli, or goji berries.

I take some vitamin supplements, for bones, for joints, for antioxidants. Even if I eat well, I also do work out a lot. These vitamins are like my insurance policy.

WHAT TO ORDER IN A RESTAURANT

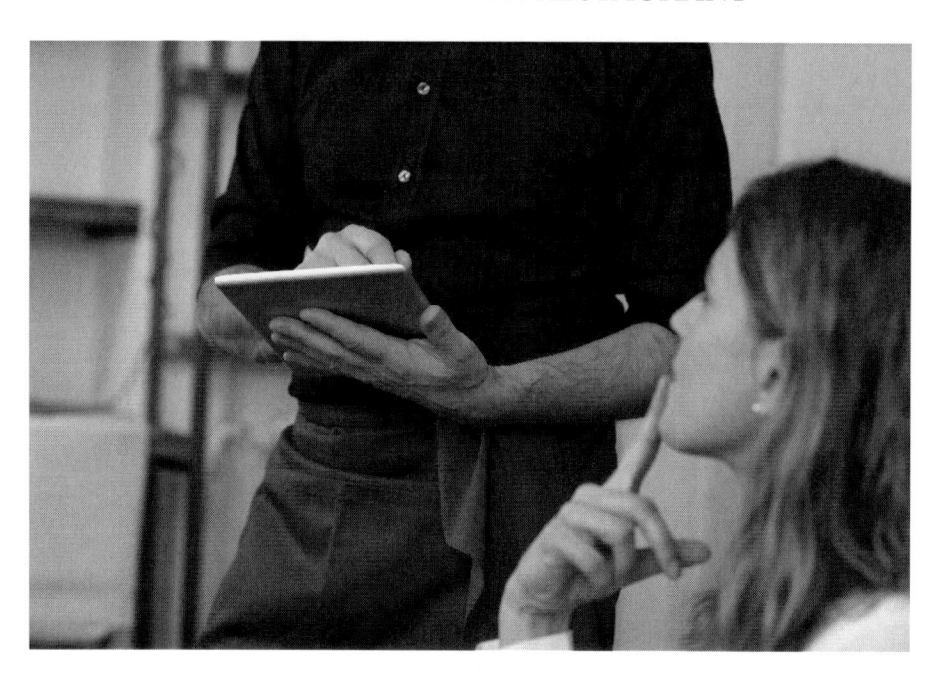

Be the person at the table that is confident enough to ask for exactly what they want, without worrying about how long it takes you to order. Take the time to ask the waiter if the chicken in the salad is deep fried or grilled. Ask if it's a creamy dressing or just oil and vinegar. Ask if there is sugar in the dressing. Ask them to put it on the side. Ask them to hold the cheese and the candied pecans. Ask them for more veggies instead of the rice with your protein. Ask them to replace the fries with a side salad, etc. You are paying for someone to make food for you. They have lots of ingredients in the kitchen, and likely, they can whip up something for you, even if it's not exactly like that on the menu.

Before you go to a restaurant, if you know in advance that you are going there, take a minute to look their menu up online and make your decision beforehand as to what you will order. You will most likely make a much better selection from home when you are not hungry, than when you are sitting in the restaurant seeing the delicious food that guests are eating around you, smelling the fantastic fragrances, feeling your stomach growling and hearing what everyone else at your table is ordering.

If you don't know in advance or if the menu is not posted online, stay strong. Repeat in your head that you are there for the company and that you will enjoy having a fantastic fun night with them without the guilt and the bloated feeling that would go along with a heavy meal.

Don't read the whole menu. Go right into the salad section, or soups and starters. Or check what are the sides for fish and meat entrees and ask for a lean protein (if you eat meat) with veggies only, no starch (skip the rice and potatoes). Find the healthiest thing on the menu and order first as soon as the waiter arrives. It will help you avoid hearing other people's tempting choices and therefore changing your mind.

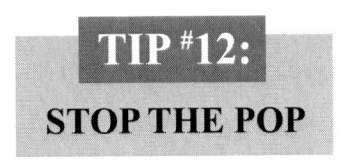

TIP #12:
STOP THE POP

12 Diet soda is better than regular.	**False** Soda = DANGER. Period.

Stop it. Now. Over. Done. That's it.

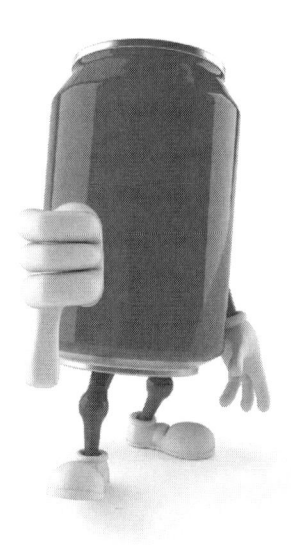

I could have mentioned it in the previous chapter. Yet, I wanted to make a point by giving it a full chapter. Not that I think that stopping soda is a skill. The skill here is to resist what people, ads, friends, are telling you about it. The skill is to change your way of seeing it. Think about it as a grenade that will sooner or later explode and create damage. Would you drink off a grenade, knowing all the damage it can create?

Pop is refined sugar. Even the diet one. Even the fruity, sparkly beverage. If it contains sugar, it is sugar. If it contains fake sugar, it is worse. On average, a can of soda contains ten teaspoons of sugar which means 40 g of sugar. Our daily intake should be 6 grams, and one pop is forty grams. (These 6 grams that we are allowed every day are very easily filled with natural sugars in fruit and healthy vegetables.) Anything that has added sugar in it should be avoided at all costs.

Start by decreasing the number of sodas you drink each week. You will get to slowly decrease the cravings of drinking that much sugar. Then eliminate it completely. In the transition, as you skip your sodas and decrease the amount you drink, if it feels too hard to have no sweet bubbly beverage in your life, mix soda water with real juice. Make sure to check the ingredients on your juice and avoid anything with added sugar. The sugar in the fruit is plenty to add a sweet flavour to your beverage.

Ideally, you can make your own soda water from your home filtered water. You can buy a machine, for example, sodastream, that makes your tap water bubbly. The device, like a soda syphon, carbonates water by adding carbon dioxide from a pressurized cylinder to create soda water (or carbonated water) to drink. I normally start by filtering my tap water in the fridge in a Brita container that is equipped with a filter to remove impurities and reduce chlorine.

By doing it yourself, it makes sure you avoid the sodium content present in the store-bought sparkling water. It even helps the environment as you are not constantly buying bottles and cans of soda water.

Stay away from the flavourings and syrup. They are just as bad as the sodas themselves. You can also just squeeze a lime or a lemon or add real fruit or cucumber to flavour it. I sometimes add some organic herbal tea leaves and let it steep in the fridge. It is not as strong as if I had plunged the herbal tea leaves in boiling water, but it is enough to give it a good flavour.

Pop is REALLY, REALLY BAD OKAY? That's it. Avoid it under all circumstances.

No more soda. Period.

TIP #13:

HAVE YOUR EXERCISE PLANNED AND STICK WITH IT... OR IMPROVISE

13 Exercising for less than thirty minutes is not worth it.	**False** This section shows you how you can be creative and find something to do every day, even if you feel that you don't have time.

YOU WILL NEVER REGRET IT

It's 6:35 am. Your alarm just went off. You are very comfortable in your sheets and somehow, your plan of getting up half an hour early to get a quick workout in before the start of your day is slowly fading. The longer you stay in bed, the more the idea of an extra half hour sleep sounds delightful.

Scenario number one. You give in to the voice telling you to go back to sleep and skip your workout. The snooze button having been pushed will nag you now every nine minutes. As you don't have to exercise anymore, you will continue to press it over and over, going back to start a new cycle of sleep every time, only to get interrupted every nine minutes. Your brain goes into a very confused mode as so many sleep cycles have been started – cycles which should last between ninety minutes to four hours. You are in a state of sleep inertia. Everything is blurry.

You finally get up at 7:30 and now realize you will be late for work. Even the shower is not enough to wake you up, and you feel rushed, you skip breakfast, apologise to your first meeting for being late and feel like you are running behind the whole day. Not only you did not get your endorphins from the exercise that you missed, you also will stay in your blurry state for most of the morning until you brain understands that you are actually up and that the snooze time was not the cue for starting a sleep cycle. Not only do you feel bad physically, but you also talk yourself down about missing your exercise. You regret not getting up. You know you would have felt so much better if you had.

Scenario number two. You fight the temptation, you get up without overthinking it (as seen in a previous chapter) and you start your day with a great sweat. You feel rejuvenated as you step out of the shower that you appreciated as a reward after your short workout. It is 7:15 am; you are ready for your day. You are not only feeling great physically, but you feel great about yourself. You are proud of having done your workout and the rest of your day unfolds brightly and positively.

You take the time for a quick, healthy breakfast and head off to work. You encounter challenges with a project, and somehow, your response to what is happening is very positive as you control your emotions and the state of mind you choose to be in, no matter the external pressure around you.

You are so proud of yourself for exercising in the morning, and you even get reinforced every time you happen to drop the line: "I got up at 6:30 am this morning to workout". You don't regret getting up.

You will never regret doing it. However, you will always regret not doing it.

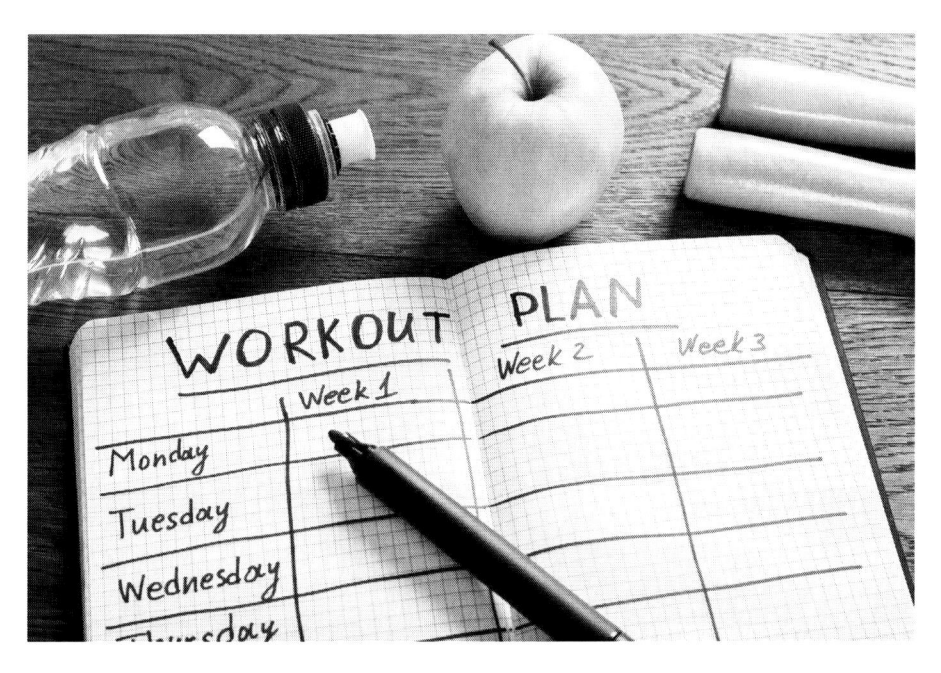

Always know in advance what will be your exercise of the day. Plan your weekly workout diligently. Make a schedule of all the moments you will reserve for exercising. Find something to do every day. Even if it is just for ten to fifteen minutes. You can always go for a walk. You can always choose to park your car four blocks away so that you get to walk for ten minutes to get to where you are going.

Make sure you include some more extended exercise, like maybe three cardio or dance classes per week, or a few strength training sessions perhaps with a personal trainer. Or perhaps on your own at home for ten to fifteen minutes, you could do a few flexibility workouts like yoga, stretching, etc. I love yoga as it counts for my flexibility and my strength at the same time. You could do ten minutes of weight lifting, then go for a twenty-minute run or power walk and do ten minutes of stretching when you get back. That is forty minutes in total. Or you can do them separately on different days.

My husband has a twenty-minute workout that he does every single morning that combines stretch and strength exercises. He does it every day even before going to teach his spin class or before going for a run. It is just on top of whatever he does.

I teach three cardio-dance classes per week, two high intensity interval training classes per week, and I run 35 to 40 minutes once or twice a week. Also, I lift weights once or twice (which is usually just before I run). After every exercise, I stretch. As I am writing this book, I don't have a yoga class on my teaching schedule, but I usually teach one yoga class per week too.

MY TWENTY MINUTE WEIGHT ROUTINE

I am very basic when it comes to what I do to keep my body toned. I do a lot of cardio and interval training in my fitness classes, along with lots of squats, burpees and push-ups in my Monday and Wednesday classes. My home workout routine is therefore very basic just to target specific muscles.

I alternate two muscle groups and usually do 2 or 3 sets of each. For example, I do a squat/lunge combo, then a combo with biceps/triceps a few times, then I would do a combo with a back exercise (like row or chin up /and a chest exercise (like a push-up or a chest press), then I would alternate abs and oblique exercise.

If I don't have much time, I simply do each muscle group once, choosing one exercise per category.

Choose a weight that is challenging for you so that the last two reps will feel hard to perform. If the weight feels too light you won't get the benefit of the exercise. If the weight is too heavy, you will already feel challenged after the second or third repetition. In that case you will not get the benefit of the exercise either because your form will more likely be compromised if the weight is too heavy for you. If you want to work in endurance and tone, you want to do 8 to 16 repetitions with a smaller weight. If you want to work for volume and bulk up, you want to do 5 to 8 repetitions with a bigger weight. In both cases, the last two repetitions should feel like you could not do any more.

BICEPS CURLS

From a standing position, holding the weights down on each side of your body, feet hip-width apart, shoulders back, chest up, pulling your stomach in to hold a strong posture, lift the weights up, bending at the elbow, keeping your elbows pointing down, squeezing your biceps on the way up and resisting on the way down.

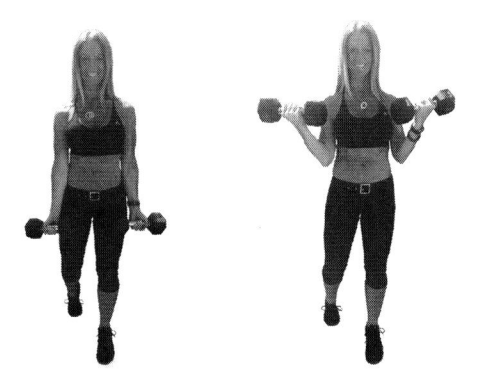

TRICEPS EXTENSION

On your back on a bench or the floor, knees bent to facilitate a flat back against the bench or the floor, keeping your abdominals engaged pulling your navel towards your spine, start with the weight overhead and bend it towards your forehead, keeping your elbows pulling towards each other to feel the tension in the triceps.

You can also do this same motion from a standing position, holding the weight overhead and keeping your elbows pointing to the ceiling.

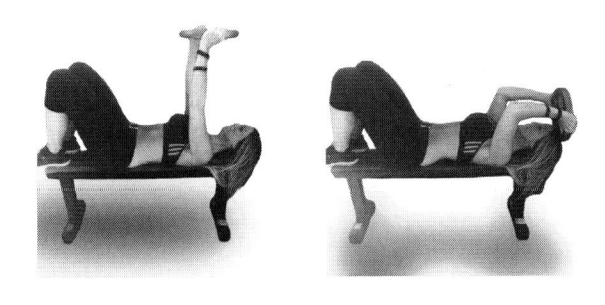

TRICEPS EXTENSION

You can do triceps extension using one single weight to really mobilize one arm at a time. Start with your elbows in line with your spine, then extend towards the back so that the top part of your arm stays still and the lower part pushes back.

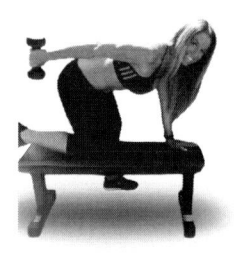

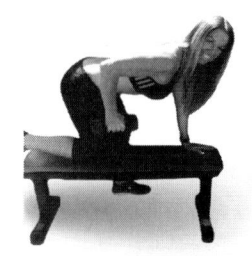

TRICEPS DIP

Start sitting on a bench or chair with your hands on each side of your body. Lower your butt towards the floor, bending your elbows so that they point towards the back, squeezing your shoulder blades together and keeping your shoulders away from your ears.

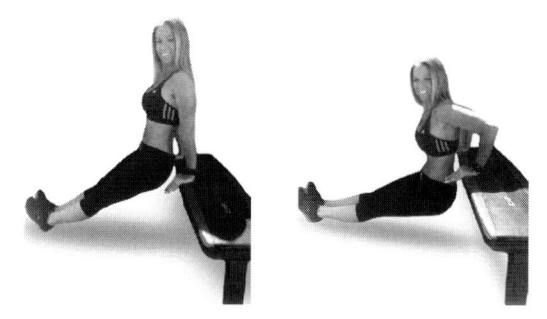

NARROW ROW - BACK

Feet hip distance apart with knees bent and bending at the waist, start with the weights down on each side of your body. Pull them up in a rowing motion with your arms close to your body.

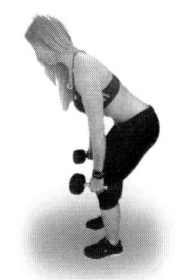

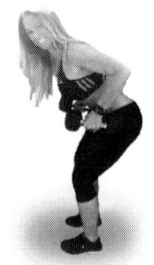

WIDE ROW - BACK

Feet hip distance apart, start with the weights down alongside your body and lift the weights up, elbows to ceiling, squeezing your shoulder blades together to work upper back.

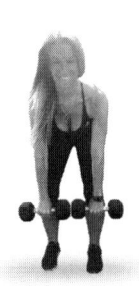

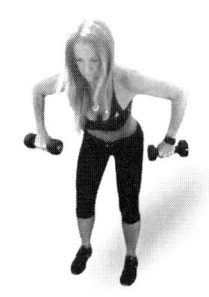

CHEST PRESS

On your back with the weights up, hands in line with your shoulders, lower the weights down with your elbows wide, then press them back up, squeezing your chest.

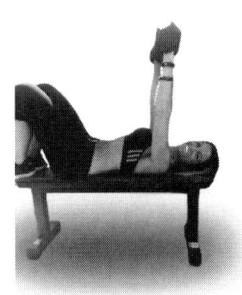

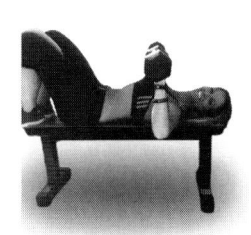

SQUAT

Feet hip distance apart, bend your knees, push your butt back, keeping the weight in your heels, pulling your belly in and keeping the chest up.

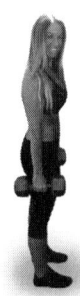

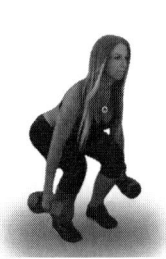

WIDE PUSH-UP – CHEST & SHOULDERS

From a plank position with your arms wide, on each side of your chest (not your face), lower yourself towards the floor and check that your elbows are forming a 90 degrees angle at the bottom of your motion. Keep your abdominals in and your shoulder blades squeezing together. Make sure you don't go down with your face between your hands, this would more likely hurt your shoulders instead of working your chest. Keep your chest between your hands. You can do the same exercise on your knees.

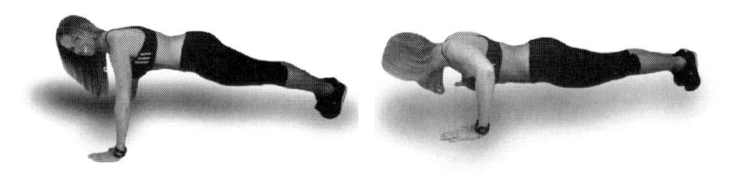

DECLINE PUSH-UP – CHEST & SHOULDERS

Same exercise as the wide push-up except that you use a bench so that your feet are higher than your upper body.

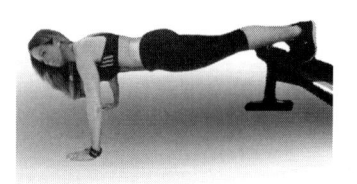

TRICEPS PUSH-UP – CHEST & TRICEPS

From a plank position with narrow hands just under the shoulders, lower yourself down so that your hands are just by your ribs at the bottom. Keep your elbows up, so that your arms are squeezing alongside your body. You can do the same exercise on your knees.

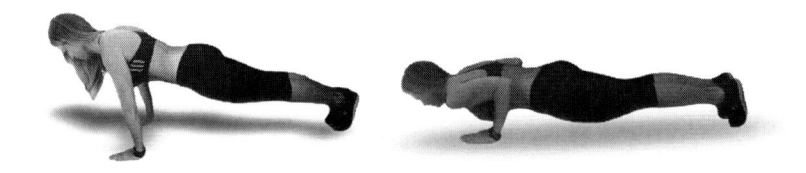

LASER WIRE PUSH-UP – CHEST & SHOULDERS

From a downward dog position, pretend that there is a laser wire right in front of you and that you have to get under. Dive under the wire, head first and then come up on the other side, pressing through your hands. Return to original position by pressing in your hands. You can do the same movement on your knees, starting from a "child's pose", knees wide, feet together, sitting back on your bum.

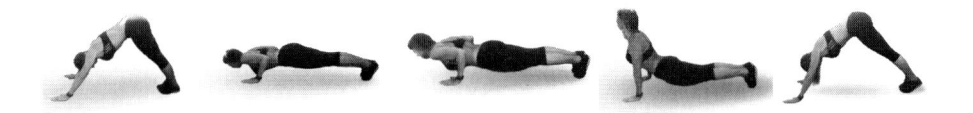

ABDOMINALS

Start with the ball between your feet. Lift your shoulders off the floor to reach towards the ball. Open up, squeezing your abdominals in to keep your back against the mat. Lower towards the floor with the ball between your legs. Come back up, lift your upper body to grab the ball in your hands. Repeat the lengthening motion, this time, with the ball between your hands. Come back up and pass the ball to your feet and repeat. You can do the same with your knees bent. You can do the same exercise without the ball.

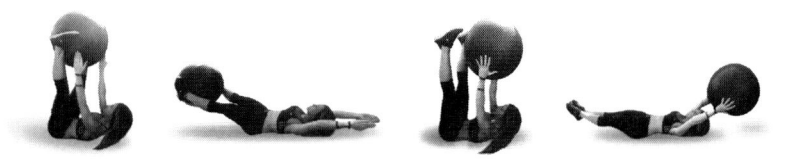

OBLIQUES

Lay sideways on a stability ball with your feet against the wall. The foot that is on top, goes to the back. Crunch sideways to lower your body against the side of the ball and crunch back up squeezing your oblique muscles. If you don't have a stability ball, you can use the couch.

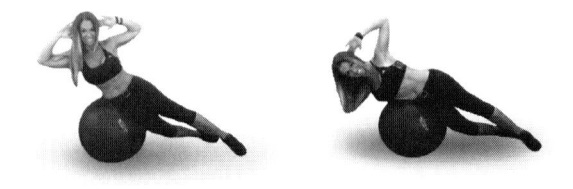

SINGLE LEG ROW

From standing with one heavy weight (double what you would use for biceps, as your legs are much stronger than your arms), lean forward, hinging at the hip, lowering the weight towards the floor as your lift your leg parallel with the floor. (Same leg as the hand holding the weight). Switch legs.

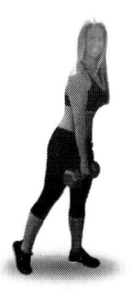

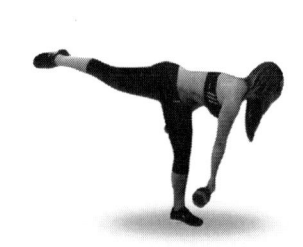

SINGLE LEG LUNGE

You can do a simple lunge with our without weights in your hands. I choose to have one foot on a stability ball to add a core functionality to the exercise. Start with a wide stance so that when you will be at the bottom of your lunge, as you roll the ball backwards, the front knee will be in line with your foot.

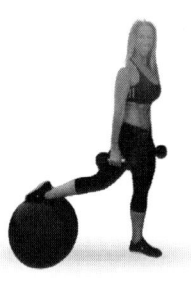

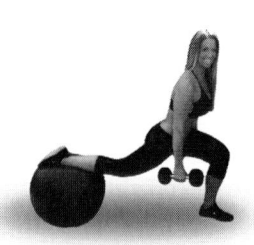

CHIN-UPS – BACK & BICEPS

I like this exercise to work my back, however, I cannot quite perform chin-ups like I used to, when I was at the top of my fitness level in my younger years. I use a band around my knee which gives me momentum to get back up. You can use underhand or overhand grip (I usually alternate one set of each).

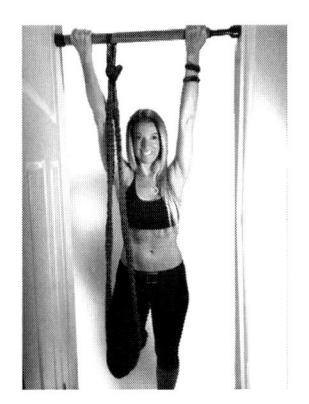

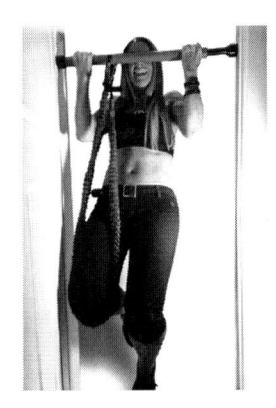

MY TEN-MINUTE HOTEL WORKOUT

I travel a lot for speaking engagements and spend lots of time in hotel rooms. At home, I have adopted the habit of going to bed early. However, when I am on the road, I often have engagements until later than I would have chosen, or I have dinners after or early starts that make my sleep time shorter than what I usually get. Therefore, that lowers my desire to set the alarm for an hour earlier in the morning to have time to exercise. My 'hotel exercise' is quite simple and only takes ten minutes. And it can take five depending on the hotel or how much time I have.

The first step is like the Friday morning routine mentioned in the "prepare your clothes in advance" chapter earlier. I prepare my clothes in advance and my shake the night before. As soon as I am dressed, the workout consists of getting out of my room, from whichever floor I am on, and take the stairs all the way down to the lobby, then turn around and go all the way up to the highest level, then walk back down to my floor. If I have time and feel like it, I do it twice or even three times when hotels have fewer storeys. Ten or so minutes later, I am in the shower and already had an excellent start to my day. With time, I can now run up the stairs, and the wheezing has diminished.

HOLIDAY WORKOUT

Let's say you are registered for a fitness class or have a personal trainer, three days per week, what happens to your training on long weekends? Do you still exercise? Your health doesn't take time off. If the class you are signed up for is cancelled on Good Friday or Labour Day Monday, call a few friends in advance and arrange to go for a walk at a specific time.

If you go for a week or two somewhere warm, pack your workout gear and make sure you have a plan to exercise while there. Most resorts are fully equipped with gyms. You can choose to use them, or you can do what my husband and I do on the beach. We go early in the morning so that we get the sweat out of the way early in the day and the sun is not as hot.

Our beach workout includes walking or a light jog on the beach for five minutes to warm up. Then we grab a lounge chair that we use as a prop for our strength and cardio exercise. We race on the beach dragging a chair behind us. We do some partners exercises too. We do abdominal crunches either on the chair or the sand. Decline push-ups, with our hands in the sand and the feet on the chair. We always bring bands with us too, which are easy to carry so we can do more biceps, triceps, shoulders, chest presses, etc.

TIP #14:
KNOW WHAT TO EAT BEFORE AND AFTER YOU TRAIN

14 You should not eat before a workout.	False Read this chapter if you are the type of person that shows up to a workout on an empty stomach.

One skill you want to become good at is to know what to eat and when to eat it.

How do you battle hunger after a workout if you're trying to lose weight? It can be difficult to lose body fat when you are trying to keep up the energy to fulfil your weekly training commitments.

Have you ever experienced substantial after-workout hunger? **Being prepared is the key.** Always know what will be your after-work-out snack and prepare it in advance. Carry it in your gym bag. Otherwise, you will get out of the gym and won't even make it home. The hunger will attack you, and you will grab anything (good or bad) that presents itself to you.

Another thing to know about is the gym reward syndrome: You feel as if you are allowed a reward for working out. You just burned 400 calories, so you might as well get that fancy coffee with whipped cream and a shot of vanilla and that danish right? And 800 calories later, you are 'up' 400 calories *after* your workout. If you had not worked out, you wouldn't have allowed the stuff you put in your mouth after.

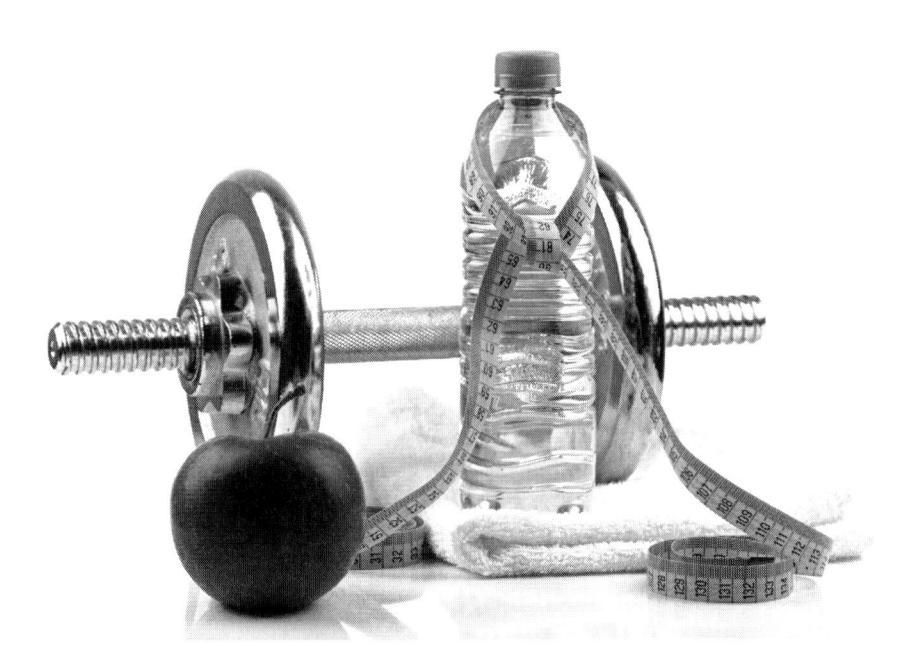

Be careful not to undo with food everything you work so hard for at the gym. I often hear that from participants in my classes: I have been coming to the gym for months. I feel that I am getting stronger but am not losing weight or fat. If that sounds like you, look carefully at your gym reward syndrome.

WHAT TO EAT BEFORE TRAINING

Avoid solid food for at least one hour before any class, or two hours before a mid to high-impact cardio class. If you're exercising early in the morning, you may not be able to eat two hours before your workout. In that case, drink something before the class such as a clean electrolyte drink with no sugar added, such as coconut water, or a shake.

Sports drinks contain sodium, which stimulates absorption and decreases urine output. Together, these effects encourage better re-hydration than water alone. However, they are often sweetened with worse ingredients than sugar, counteracting the benefit you would get from them. Remember to make sure they are made with good, clean ingredients. I use coconut water. Unlike most sports drinks, it is natural and clean. Again, *read the labels!*

Bananas work for me in the morning before a workout. I usually make a half a banana shake with my protein powder and water.

If you work out at 6 p.m., you should have a snack around 4 p.m. Have a low glycemic index meal–the type of carbohydrates that produce only small fluctuations in our blood glucose and insulin levels–before endurance exercise. It will improve your performance. Avoid high-fat meals because fat slows down the digestion and stomach-emptying process.

Try to stick to moderate fibre and protein, for example:

- Avocado
- Hard-boiled egg
- Water smoothie with fruit
- Plain yoghurt with fresh fruit
- Rice cakes with nut butter or salsa

WHAT TO EAT WHILE TRAINING

Water, water, water! Water is the best drink, certainly before exercise and during exercise of fewer than ninety minutes. If exercising more than ninety minutes, or if you tend to sweat heavily, then an electrolyte drink may be a good idea for you.

WHAT TO EAT AFTER TRAINING

Remember two things:

- Within <u>thirty minutes</u> of your workout, you must have carbohydrates. Carry something with you to make sure you replenish—a piece of fruit or something to get those carbs in fast within the thirty minutes. I carry dates with me in my gym bag. Muscle tissue is like a sponge, with big holes, and it's wide open right after your workout. You need to fill the holes (with carbs) right afterwards, or the next exercise will feel 'crunchy'. The muscles just won't work as well. Just like a dry sponge.

- Within <u>two hours</u> after strength training, and sometimes after cardio, you need to eat protein. I choose a hard-boiled egg or quinoa (both in my salad), or beans in my soup, as these are the main proteins in my diet. A nut butter toast also does the trick.

PART 5:
BELIEFS AND VALUES

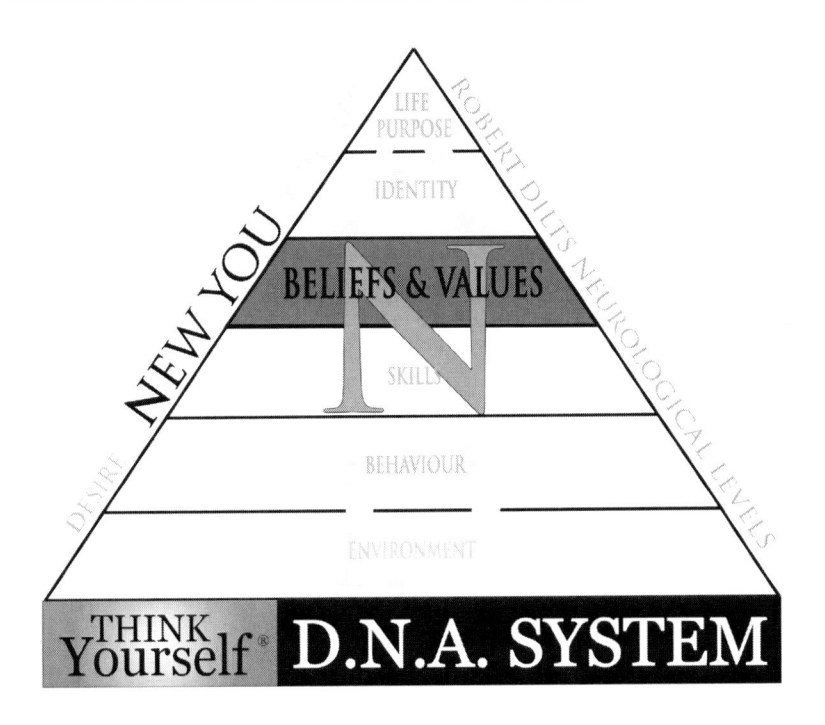

Pyramid diagram: Robert Dilts' Neurological Levels — from top to bottom: LIFE PURPOSE, IDENTITY, BELIEFS & VALUES, SKILLS, BEHAVIOUR, ENVIRONMENT. Labeled "NEW YOU" and "DESIRE" on the sides, with "Think Yourself® D.N.A. SYSTEM" at the base.

A belief is what you believe is true, in your own representational systems, and is forming who you are. Beliefs are at the base of our habits (good or bad). We need to change our old negative beliefs in order to replace them with beliefs that will serve us better.

You will know you have stepped into the sticky realm of beliefs and values if you find yourself saying: "I just keep doing that thing I said I wasn't going to do." Your choices defy logic as your unconscious mind rules. You feel like an ant plugging away in one direction, one step at a time, doing everything you can towards your goal and you don't realize that the ant is walking on the back of an elephant that is walking in the opposite direction.

The ant can go as fast as she can, but the elephant is exponentially so much bigger that, even in her best efforts, she will never counteract the direction the elephant is going towards. That is why we sometimes feel that we self-sabotage ourselves. Our unconscious mind is so much more powerful, that even if logically we try to adopt new serving habits and behaviours, if our unconscious mind is not on board, like the elephant, it will take us in the opposite direction.

Somehow, you feel that you are doing everything right and plugging away with your behaviours and skills. But your dedicated steps toward your goal will be in vain, if your beliefs and values are going in the opposite direction.

Most people's problems reside in the beliefs and values level. The closer to the identity level at the top, the more you see it as a real problem. An easy example of this is when someone has a self-confidence problem (belief) and to give themselves some more prestige and power, they buy an expensive sports car. The problem is in the belief level (self-confidence) and they are trying to fix it at the environment level (sports car). It can't work. Again, the problem needs to be addressed where it belongs.

I am not saying that all the tips that I gave you so far don't work. They do. Yet, the most important ones are yet to come. If you don't change your beliefs, all the tips in the world, even applied to the letter, will not do anything for you.

Our beliefs and values are guiding all our actions. When they make us grow and give us fulfilling lives, we can thank them for making life easy for us. When, on the other hand, they make us see the world from a negative angle, we wish we could change them. The beliefs that are not serving us are called *limiting beliefs.*

We have seen in behaviours, that most of the time, the problem is with the values or beliefs layer and cannot be fixed at the behavioural level. If a problem resides in the identity or the belief system of a person, that is where the problem needs to be addressed. This explains why some of the past attempts at losing weight failed. It is because it was not addressed at the right level. If you believe you are overweight (beliefs and values level) then exercising and eating well (both behaviours) will not fix the problem. You will keep self-sabotaging yourself until you correct the beliefs.

TIP #15:
CATCH WHAT YOU SAY & THINK

| **15** Affirmations don't work. | **True** Affirmations will have no impact if they are not well formed and don't 'feel' true when you say them out loud. |

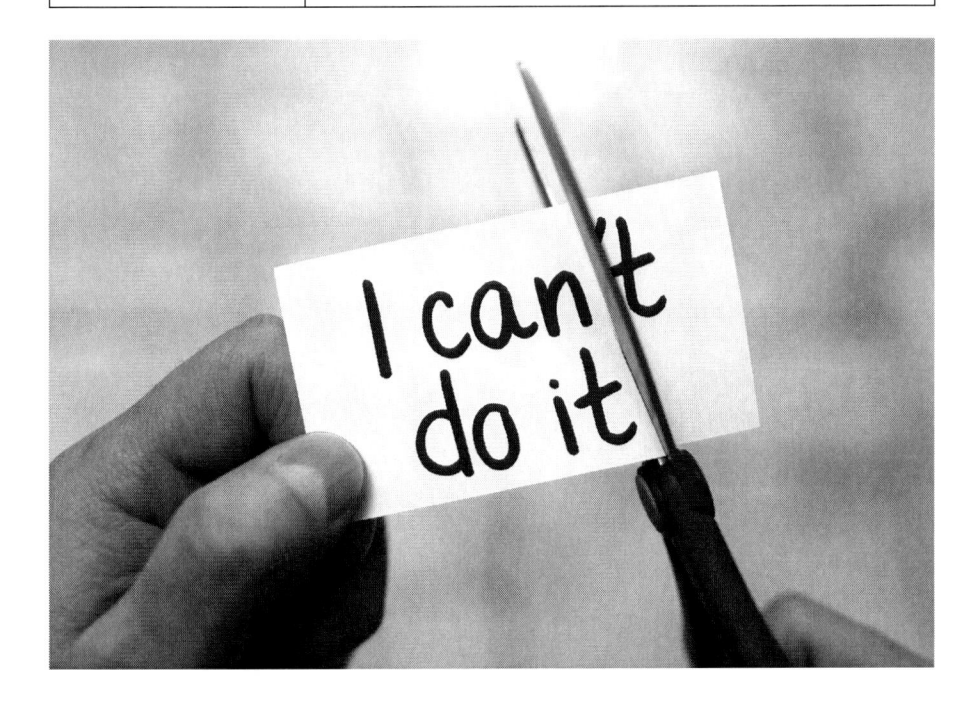

Your priority from now on is to listen to what you say and think. Start catching your thoughts and immediately rephrase them if you judge that they are not serving you. You will quickly become very good at it.

More likely, if you believe that being healthy is hard, then you are telling your brain and programming it to make it difficult for you. Every time you think about health, you are giving a reason for your brain to make it hard for you.

Have you ever heard yourself say: "No matter how hard I work or what I do, I can't get healthy." Have you ever thought that this belief, and its constant repetition in your head, might be the main reason that has kept you from getting healthy all these years?

When you rephrase an affirmation, you have to make sure that it feels right when you say it out loud. If the voice inside your head says: "Yeah, right, totally untrue", then the affirmation is not well phrased. Find a way to change the affirmation until it sits well with you and that you feel that it is believable.

Some rephrasing examples:

> As I am working on my diet, I am getting healthier every day.
> I can feel progress with my health as I am working towards it.
> I am in the process of getting healthy and fit.
> I am on my way to my ideal weight. It's working.

Here is another common limiting belief: "I don't have Willpower".

You can't be buying every single junk food at the grocery store. You more likely walk past hundreds of unhealthy treats every time you shop. Somehow, you do have willpower for these. You do avoid a lot of unhealthy behaviours daily. You do have willpower for that. You get up in the morning, you show up to work, somehow. You have willpower for that too. It is inside you. You got it. You can apply it to anything you want. The problem is that for some specific foods, we have given ourselves permission to succumb. You have programmed yourself to be weak in the presence of the said temptation. Believing that certain foods like chocolate, pastries, chips, etc. have control over you is not serving you. You want to catch these thoughts and start rephrasing them right away, as soon as you become aware of them.

Repeat phrases like:

> I have control over what I eat.
> I nourish myself with healthy food.
> I am willing to learn how it feels to have control over food.
> I am in the process of choosing healthy food to nourish my body.

Here is another example of a limiting belief: "Being healthy is a lot of work".

Firstly, what is more work? Being healthy or unhealthy? When I look at unhealthy people, I can't help but appreciate how amazing it feels to have my health. I am so grateful for being able to run to the store quickly and come back with heavy bags, thinking nothing of it. I am so grateful that I get to do whatever I want and never have to cancel plans because I am not feeling great. My heart is strong, and my immune system is bullet-proofing me against a virus that everyone around me seems to catch but me.

The fruit and veggies and antioxidants that I abundantly nourish myself with make my skin glow and my hair shine so that I don't have to spend a fortune or an enormous amount of time on make-up and hair products. I am thankful for not having to replace my favourite clothes every season because I outgrew them. I can wear whatever I want, and I am always sure it will fit me. When I go out to an event, I can choose my favourite dress, without worrying about being able to get into it. When I play with our grandson, I can run almost as fast as him and I can keep up with his active lifestyle. I can have a long day of presenting conferences for four to six hours of standing, and still have energy at the end of the day for socializing. I think that being healthy makes everything so much easier. It is actually the reverse. Being unhealthy is a lot of work.

You can start rephrasing your belief with:

> Being healthy is rewarding.
>
> Being healthy is worth it.
>
> Being healthy makes my life easy.
>
> I am in the process of making being healthy easier.
>
> I am willing to learn how it feels to think that being healthy is easy.
>
> I am changing my normal so that being healthy becomes easy.

TIP #16:
YOU DON'T NEED TO FEEL FULL

16 You need your food to be satisfying	**False** This chapter breaks down the belief that we need to feel full after a meal.

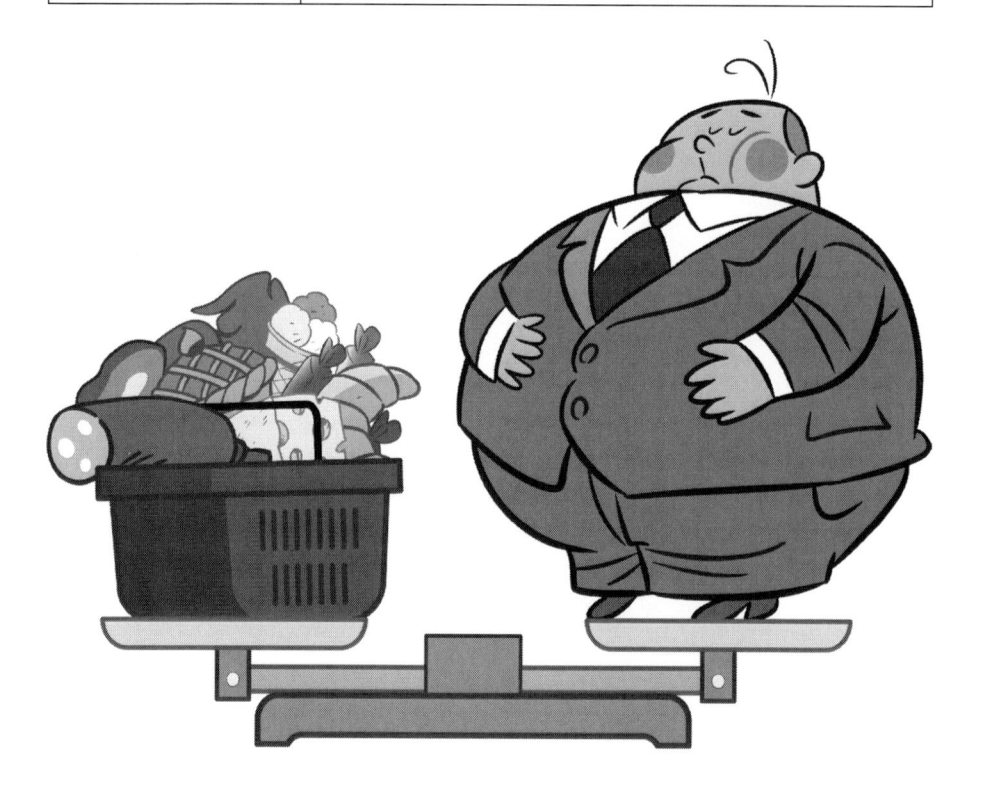

My husband once asked me to help him find something that could replace his bread. He was trying to shed a few pounds and he thought that letting go of bread was a good strategy. Bread in itself can be healthy. There are great options. There are sprouted grains, thin slices, whole flour, gluten-free, etc. In itself, bread is not causing us to be unhealthy or overweight. The two main problems with bread are the fact that we may eat too much of it, and the fact that it is often a vehicle for foods that are not so healthy or high in calories.

It is very common to find the following on top of toast: butter, coconut oil, Nutella, jam, peanut butter, almond butter, cheese, etc. Even if some of these options are healthy, like the coconut oil and the almond butter, we are very often surpassing the recommended portion size. One or two tablespoons is all we should use. If you think about how thick you spread your favourite things on your bread, you more than likely have way too much of it.

Knowing this, how he puts way too much nut butter or cheese on his toast (of which a portion size should be a pink eraser) and acknowledging that he was going way overboard with this 'vehicle' for calories, my husband wanted to quit bread. He asked me to help him find something else that could fill him up. We usually eat oatmeal (steel-cut oats) in the morning– see the last chapter where I share my breakfast and tip number one on prepping food. With the oatmeal or with cereal, my husband used to like to have a piece of toast which would help him feel full. He found that just the oatmeal was not enough for him to have a 'full' feeling.

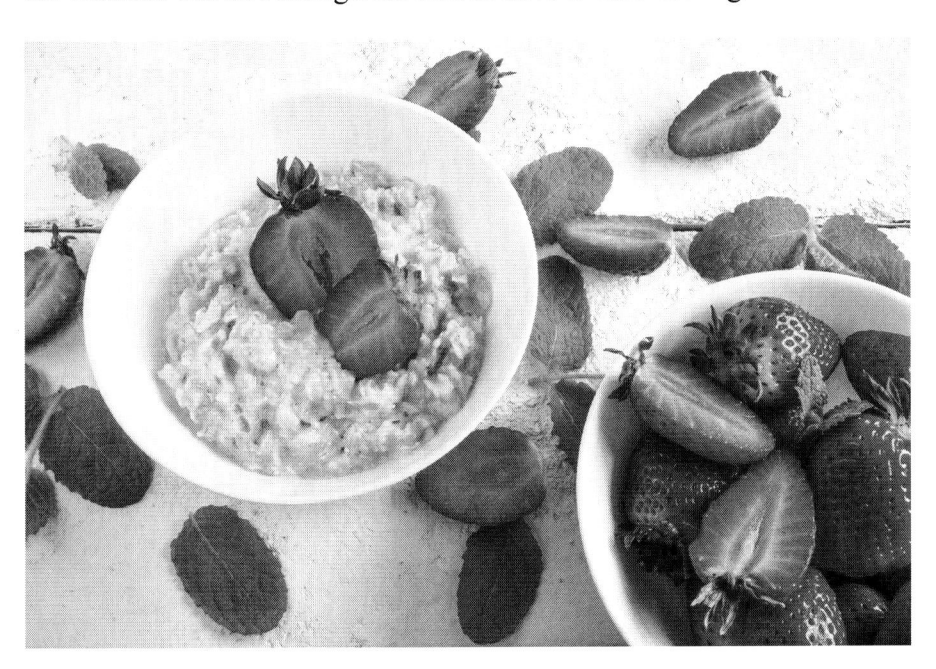

When discussing this with me, I suggested that instead of trying to find something to replace the bread, we should work on changing the limiting belief that he needed to feel full after a meal. We do have a big stomach with enough room to store food, so that our ancestors could skip even a few days before eating again as they were hunting their next prey.

In our society, it is really not necessary for us to fill up. This sensation of feeling full is actually a detriment to our health. *If you feel full, it is actually because you ate too much.* We should not be feeling full at the end of a meal. In fact, as soon as you had your first bite, you are not hungry anymore. We are only hungry when our hunger and satiety hormones are sending a signal to our brain. (See tip number six on how biology works).

Switch your plates for smaller ones and eat only one serving. You can always have a healthy snack mid-morning or mid-afternoon to keep you energised until the next meal. (See number four on snacking).

By switching his mindset, my husband was able to shed the pounds he wanted and he now eats regular portions of food without needing to feel full.

How do you get your mind on board?

Before each meal, continually repeat to yourself that you will be satisfied with the food. As soon as you eat your first bite, tell yourself that you are getting full with every bite.

CHEW

It's a great thing to do the mental work. We also need to get biology to follow. The first step of digestion starts in your mouth. You need to puree your food in your mouth by chewing completely. When you start changing your eating process, it can feel like an eternity in the beginning. If you do chew every bite patiently until it is fully pureed before you swallow, it will help your digestion considerably and slow down your eating process. This will allow some time for your satiety hormones to have time to travel from your stomach to your brain in order to send you the message that you can stop eating now because you are full. (See tip number six on making sure you are fed.)

Chewing is a wonderful thing. I went for blood tests once at my Naturopathic doctor and he explained to me that some softer foods, easy to swallow without proper chewing, show up a lot in the bloodstream when doing allergy tests. Nowadays, most people who get tested come back with eggs, wheat, etc. in the list of food they have a 'sensitivity' for. It may be true. Or as the doctor explained to me, it may simply be that the person did not chew their food enough.

When you don't chew, your food is not fully absorbed by your cells to give them the nutrients. Therefore, this food can show up in your blood test, just like if you were allergic to it. Most people are not. They are just not chewing enough. Think about it, when you eat an egg, which is soft and easy to swallow, a few bites will do the trick for it to pass through your throat, right? But it still won't digest properly. You want your food to go through every single step of the digestion process, which starts in your mouth. If you skip a step, just because it is a soft food, you will require much longer to digest it and risk not being able to digest it completely. You want your food to be used as energy. You don't want it to simply be causing you heartburn all day.

Since this explanation from my Naturopathic doctor, I have been chewing forever before swallowing my food. Not only does it allow me to feel full faster, causing me to eat less and ingest fewer calories, it also helps me to digest easier, avoiding some foods being stored in unwanted areas.

EAT NUTS

I have mentioned this a few times already. Here is more on the nuts subject. If you are gaining weight because your portions are too big, eating nuts will help you lose weight. Here's how. There is good fat in a nut, which sends a signal to your brain that tells you you're full. (You have read the full biological reaction explained in tip number six). It takes about twenty minutes for the signal to make it to your brain. Eat a few nuts about twenty minutes before your meal; it will send a signal to your brain that you're full by the time you start eating. You'll keep your portions smaller. How much are a few nuts? A handful. Whatever doesn't fit in your hand is too many.

TIP #17:

RECOGNIZE WHEN IT'S JUST A SCRATCH

17 When you make a bad choice, nutrition-wise, you should keep going as your day is a write-off anyways. You will start fresh the following day.	False You will learn in the upcoming chapter how to interrupt the pattern when something goes sideways.

There is a common tendency to overindulge once the 'health-seal' has been broken. Do you sometimes eat very healthfully, you are on a roll, you are doing everything right and then, here it is, the amazing decadent chocolate fudge cupcake, staring at you with its sumptuous icing, working all inches of your willpower until you finally give in and buy it. You run to your car and eat it quickly before anyone can see you and you are not even finished enjoying yourself when the guilt has already started to eat you alive. You know that cupcakes are unhealthy, and you now think that your whole day, or week, of healthy choices just went to waste.

WHAT YOU HEAR

You think of yourself as a loser, and you are really down on yourself for your lack of willpower. You keep saying to yourself: "Well, of course, I bought the cupcake, I am very weak". "I have a sweet tooth, what can you do?" "Now my whole day is a wreck. I might as well eat another one right now and also have a burger and fries for dinner." And more likely, you will also have dessert for dinner too because your day is screwed up anyways.

WHAT YOU DO

You proceed to go back in and buy another cupcake, or you stop at the coffee shop drive-thru to get a doughnut, or at the gas station to buy a chocolate bar and a tub of ice cream for dessert. If you're going to 'fail' your day, you want to do it big!

WHAT IT IS LIKE

This whole scenario is like stomping on your phone because you accidentally dropped it and made a little scratch on the screen. Your phone is perfectly fine. The scratch is actually barely perceptible. And yet, as you see what you have done in dropping your phone, you would put it back on the floor and start stomping on it to 'finish it off'.

WHAT TO SAY INSTEAD

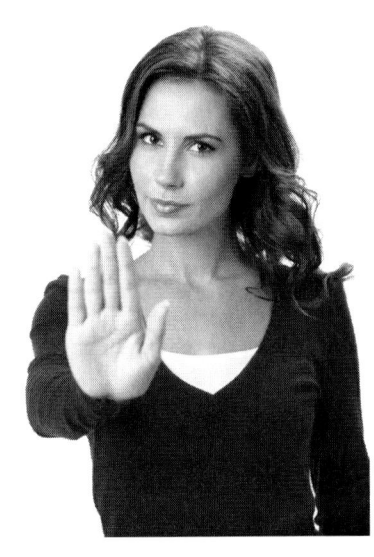

Stop the bleeding. When eating something you should not have or doing the reverse of what you know you should be doing, like sitting on the couch instead of going for your workout, we tend to be really hard on ourselves. This sends negative messages to our personal assistant (see section one on how your personal assistant can work on your side).

You want to immediately say things like: "Hmm, this tastes great, and I know it is not so healthy for me, so that is why I very rarely eat this." "This is a 'one-off'", "I am usually awesome at making great choices", "I always eat very healthy", "I will catch up for the rest of the day and make sure I have proper nutrition from now on."

Or, "This was actually tasting pretty off, especially from the second bite on, I enjoy healthy food much more than this."

TIP #18:
GET PERMANENT WITH IT

18 When you lose weight, you always gain it back.	**False** This a very common limiting belief that needs to go.

Some people are very diligent in doing everything right to lose weight. They even note everything so that when they gain the weight back, they will have everything recorded so that they know exactly how they lost it so that they can start over. Somehow, we are programmed for our weight loss to be temporary. We believe that the weight will come back. Interestingly enough, it does. Not because it is the reality, but because it is our belief about reality.

Changing this belief is key in order to make your weight loss efforts temporary and your new weight permanent. It is like you have your own thermostat set at a specific temperature. If for some reason, the temperature gets colder or warmer, your thermostat will sense it and will work behind the scenes to re-establish the set temperature.

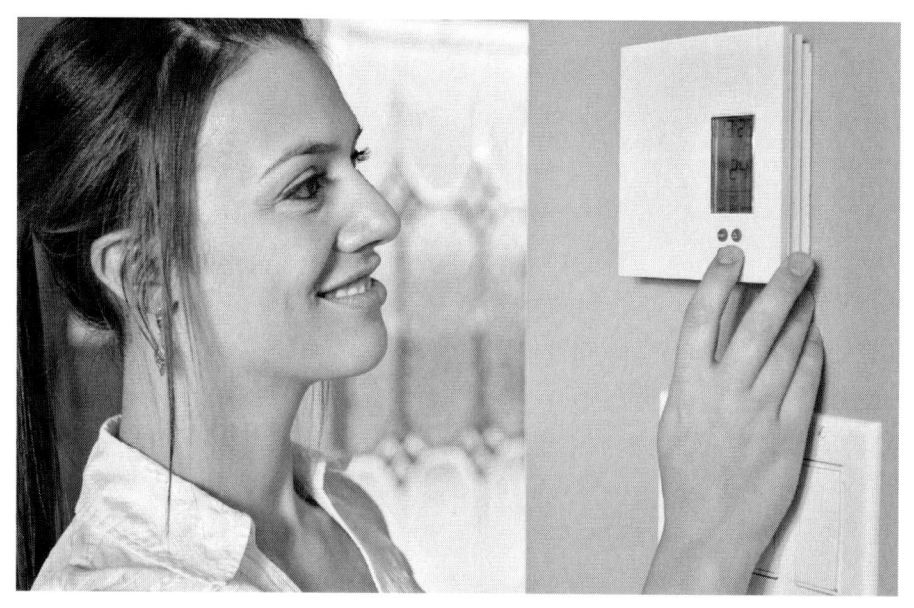

After having kids, or after moving to a different city or after quitting hockey three times per week, you may have gained weight. Somehow, your brain has accepted this new weight to be your new standard. Refuse it. Decide what you want your normal to be and get back there. Reset your thermostat. Adjust it to the weight you want and create a compelling image in your head about this being the weight that you will now have for the rest of your life. Remember how it felt to be this size. What people told you. What you were saying to yourself in your head when you were in that great shape. If you cannot remember a time when you were smaller than you are now, create a new movie in your head of how it would look like and feel like.

Change your belief to:

I am on my way to go back to my normal weight.

I am resetting my new normal to my ideal weight.

I am willing to feel how it feels to love my body and myself.

TIP #19:
HAVE HEALTHY THINGS TO MAKE YOU FEEL GREAT

19 Food makes us feel good.	True This chapter explains the emotional connections we have with food.

It is 11 a.m. on a Saturday morning. Peak time in a busy grocery store. You are two years old. Somehow you haven't had a full night, and you are pretty irritable. As you and your mother are lining up for the next available cashier, your mom is trying to control your temper tantrum getting louder and louder until you eventually start to yell as loud as you can in a cry that nobody can ignore. Your mom loves you very much. She would do anything for you. She is embarrassed by everyone staring at her in the grocery store and at this point, she would do anything to make you quiet.

She uses a tactic that her own mom used on her, successfully, when she was kid.

She says: "If you can stay quiet for a few more minutes until we finish paying, we will go for ice cream after." To any kid, the idea of ice cream is usually enough to motivate them to stop the scene and calm down. When this happens, you actually start feeling better. The idea of a sweet treat makes you forget the reason you were unhappy in the first place, and it moves you to a different state.

Unfortunately, your brain associates the ice cream, or sweet treat, with a coping mechanism that works to make you feel better. Later on in life, whenever you don't feel right, your brain reminds you of that strategy that was developed in your early years. Our parents are not bad people, and we are not either if we have used the same with our own kids. We don't realize the damage that we create in our kids' brain with this strategy.

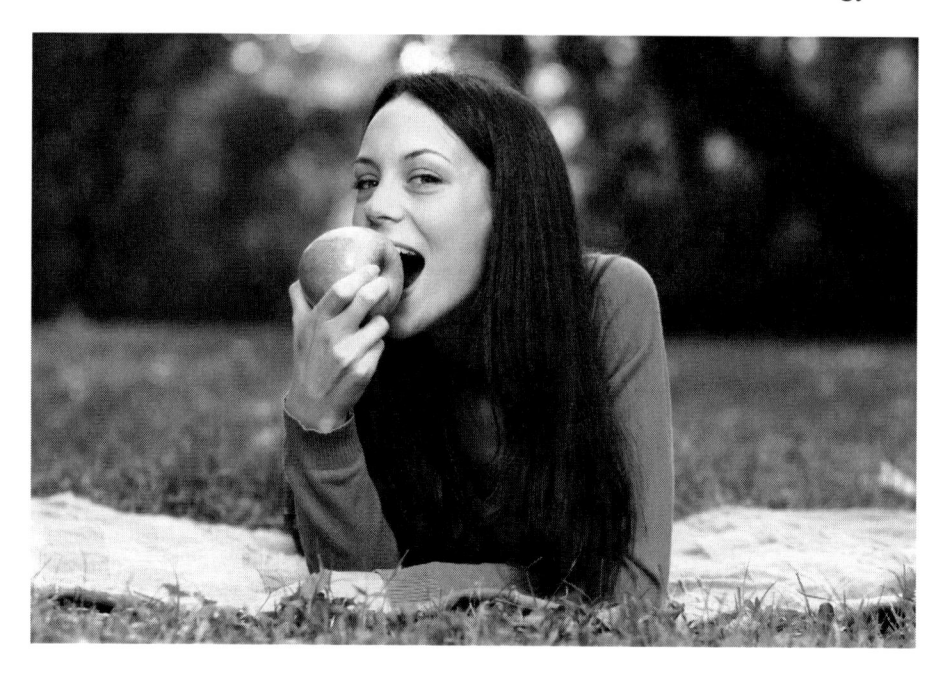

The good news is that you can reverse this. Understanding how this neural pathway was created, that the intention behind the craving of the ice cream was to feel better, you can now think of a different way that can fulfil this intention. How else, other than using a destructive behaviour, can you feel better? Going for a walk? Going to the gym? Cutting a fresh ripe mango? Sitting down in your favourite chair with a herbal tea and a book? Listening to music? Meditating? Whatever works for you, find one thing that makes you feel great and use it as your new strategy to create a new neural pathway that your brain will eventually start adopting more and more, until it becomes unconscious and natural.

FIND THE INTENTION BEHIND THE BEHAVIOUR

Remember the premise that more likely, if you are about to 'eat your emotions', it means that behind the scenes, the food is not what you want. Find the intention behind the behaviour. Once you know what it is that you are after, make up a new way to fulfill that intention.

We initially self-sabotage in order to keep us safe and in our comfort zone. Most behaviours start with good intentions. Even the teenager who takes up smoking to belong in the group, even criminals usually start out with good intentions, and then go downhill from there.

Finding the intention behind the behaviour becomes quite relevant when it comes to getting rid of a bad habit. A coaching client wanted to quit smoking. All on his own, he decreased his habit to one cigarette per day, but was unable to completely quit. It turned out—after asking the right questions during coaching sessions—that he had not yet accepted the fact that his father had passed away. His father was a smoker, so the cigarette was connecting him with memories of his father. He did not want to let him go. Finding the intention behind the unwanted behaviour helps to find other ways to fulfill that positive intention. Now, instead of having his one cigarette at night (the unwanted behaviour), he takes out the photo album and looks at photos of his father, so he can connect and honour his memory. He has been smoke-free for almost 8 years and is now running half-marathons.

Our cravings are often connected to deeper memories and triggered by our senses. We all know that certain smells remind us of certain things. Mom's cooking always made us feel good. Have you ever walked into a movie theatre or a bakery? You can smell the popcorn or the freshly baked goods, and immediately the cravings start. Find the reason behind the craving and then find a different way to fulfill that craving. If you miss your mom, call her or look at some pictures. You don't need to eat a whole chocolate cake because it makes you think about her. You can still think about her and love her without having to sabotage your health!

Here is another great example that shows how finding the intention behind the behaviour can help modify the behaviour. I had a client once who moved to a new city. Out of the blue, she kept buying a certain type of chocolate bar and devouring it, and she couldn't understand why. Every day she needed that chocolate bar. She never used to like chocolate and it was never a problem before, even when she actually worked for the manufacturer of that particular chocolate bar (which was quite ironic, a chocolate sales rep who doesn't like chocolate).

So why was she all of a sudden eating chocolate? What had changed? She called me and said: "Nathalie, you have to help me, I am eating chocolate every day and I am going out of my mind! I never used to like chocolate! What is going on?"

After a few sessions, we realized she missed the life she had working for the chocolate company. She had moved and was now alone in a new city. Eating chocolate was her way of coping with feeling lonely and missing her friends. She didn't really want the chocolate bar; she wanted to be with her old friends. Now, instead of eating chocolate bars, she phones or connects with her friends on email or Facebook, which is a much healthier way to fulfill the intention behind her behaviour. She has gotten back to her healthy eating habits and is now in Australia, but she still keeps in touch with her friends on the web.

Sometimes you can start with concrete physiological tricks to help you get an instant calming effect. Once calm and relaxed, you are then more capable to get into your deeper self and have a good discussion with yourself.

Here are a few physical things you can do to start re-wiring your brain to use healthy things to make your feel great.

BREATHE

You don't always have time to find a park to go for a walk. You can simply sit back and take a few seconds to breathe. Deeply. Slowly. Inhaling through your nose and exhaling through your mouth. Sit so your back is comfortably supported, legs uncrossed, with your hands resting ever so lightly on your thighs. Get in connection with your unconscious mind. Inside. Where everything is clear, and simple. In your mind's eye, walk the ten steps toward reaching that connection with your deeper structure. First step, inhale. Second step, exhale. Third step inhale. Fourth step exhale. Step number five, start feeling calm. Step number six, feeling relaxed. Step number seven, your mind feels really clear. Step number eight, everything seems simple. Step number nine, entering your deeper self. Step number ten, fully connected with your unconscious mind.

Take a few seconds to enjoy this time, fully calm and relaxed inside, where everything is clear and simple. You have all the answers your need. You got this. You are awesome. Stay for as long as you can and slowly walk back, fully rejuvenated. You will be amazed at how quick you can reset and center yourself.

FIND CALMING GREEN

If you don't have time to submerge yourself in nature, having plants in your office helps you induce a more relaxed state. Research from Washington State University show that a group of stressed-out people entering a room full of plants had their stress level lowered by four points.[2]

If you have the luxury of having a window, look outside to stare at green grass, flowers, plants or trees. You may have to get up and walk to the closest window to get your "green-fix". A few mindful minutes will work on making you feel great. If none of it is an option, maybe a frame with a gorgeous green outdoor scene can be your focal point on your desk.

---

2 Lohr, V.I., C.H. Pearson-Mims, and G.K. Goodwin. *Journal of Environmental Horticulture*. 14(2) "Interior plants may improve worker productivity and reduce stress in a windowless environment." 97-100. 1996.

MASSAGE YOUR HAND

You can apply pressure or massage from the base of the junction between your thumb and second finger and the base of the second and third finger, all the way up to the tips of these three fingers.

In reflexology, the tips of the thumb, pointer finger, and middle finger relate directly to your brain. Massaging the base will create an instant feeling of calmness.

MUSIC

Take a three-minute break to listen to one of your favourite songs. Calming classical music is known to calm you down; however, I find that any song that you love will do the trick, no matter the genre. Make sure it is a song that generates great feelings. For example, if you have a broken heart and you are trying to replace your emotional eating by music, don't choose a love song that will make it worse. Identify songs that make you feel good!

If you don't have headphones handy, you can sing it in your head or hum the chorus. That will have a beneficial effect.

LAUGH

Watch a viral video online, google a joke, or watch a comedy show if you are at home. Laughter is known to improve your mood increasing your endorphin level. If you can, call a fun friend and spend time doing something fun. Do something silly that will generate laughter.

TIP #20:

BE LEFT WANTING IT BEFORE THE FIRST BITE

20 Feeling that we want to eat bad stuff is wrong.	**False** This chapter is dedicated to learning to live with the desire of certain foods, instead of trying to get away from wanting them.

I remember the days when I could eat three doughnuts in a row. And I am sure I could have eaten a whole box by myself. Yes. I have been there too. The thought that is saving me now is: "I will be left wanting it anyways." Somehow, it will never be enough.

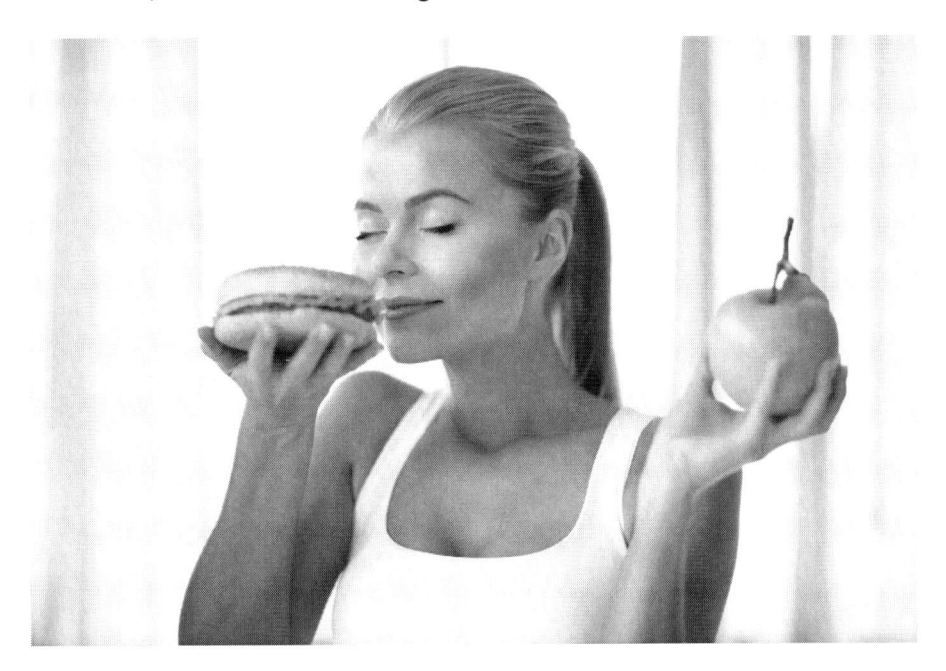

When you want to have a piece of cake or a few fries, you are, in your mind, thinking about the said attractive food. You want it. You think you even 'need' it and it somehow calls your name and haunts you. What I noticed was that once I have had a piece of cake, or a doughnut, or fries, or chips, or anything unhealthy, I am left wanting more. I need another piece, or another handful.

And now that my mouth knows what it tastes like, now that it has experienced the sweetness of the icing or the crunchiness and saltiness of the chips, it is even harder to resist. I want more. I have come to the conclusion that **if I will be left wanting another piece of cake anyway, I should be left wanting it BEFORE the first one.**

This way of thinking has tremendously helped me in changing my desires for unwanted food and allowed me to gradually change my 'normal' so that I now consider them as non-existent in my everyday diet.

PART 6:
IDENTITY

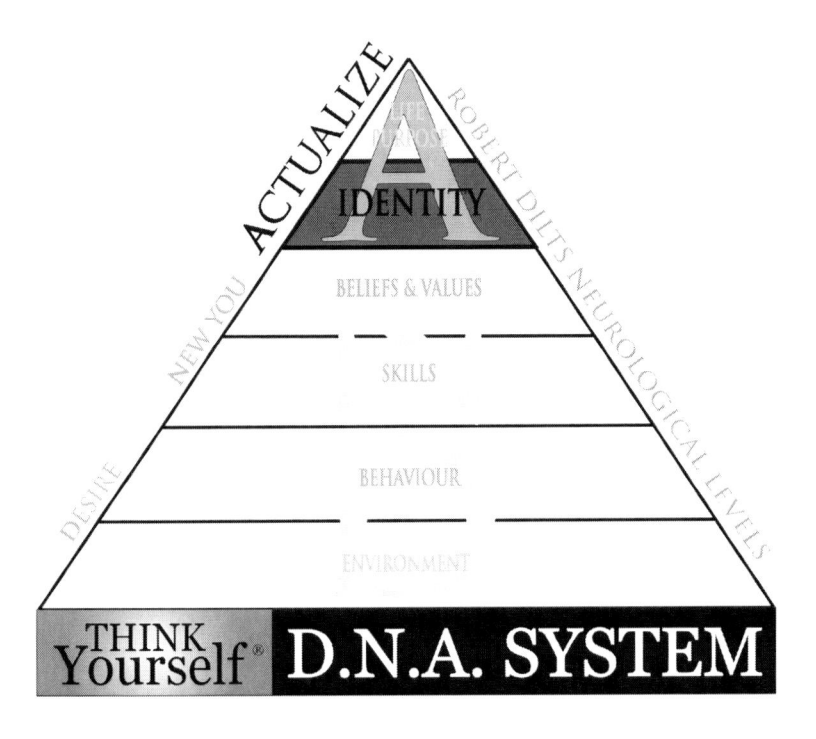

Think Yourself® D.N.A. SYSTEM

(Pyramid diagram — Robert Dilts Neurological Levels: IDENTITY / BELIEFS & VALUES / SKILLS / BEHAVIOUR / ENVIRONMENT; "ACTUALIZE" / "NEW YOU" / "DESIRE")

Our identity is who we are. Our self-esteem, our sense of self and what we identify with. It can include identifying with our job, marriage, religion, etc. It can also include how we interpret events regarding our own self-worth. What we think we deserve or not.

You may be familiar with the expression, 'I AM a morning person.' It is a deep belief about who we are at a core level. We are not born to be morning or evening people. We choose to be more effective in the morning (or not) because we think so, act so and articulate this 'fact' to others. Saying the words: 'I AM' a morning person is a symbol of a deeply ingrained belief. It is much different from saying, "I work well in the morning" or "I get up early" which are behavioural affirmations and not identity-related.

Understanding each level of our own self and identifying where the problems lie is a significant step towards fixing it. When we hear people say, "I am overweight," it's important to recognize that the words I AM are very powerful. It means they don't only think of themselves as having a few pounds to lose. They say I AM, which refers to their deeply ingrained beliefs at the level of their identity.

When we implement change, the higher we go on the neurological levels, the more profoundly we need to dig into our ingrained beliefs about ourselves to make the change. By changing cars or clothes, we are only changing an environmental aspect of our life. But by changing who we are, we lose, in some aspect, a portion of who we are.

Most people are quite wary of change, as no one wants to lose their sense of self. Who are they going to be if they cannot be who they thought they were all their life? That is when re-writing our software and deciding what and who we want to be is an empowering tool that allows us to let go of our old self and embrace our new identity.

Whenever we say to ourselves: "I am", we are referring to the *identity level,* down in our deepest structure. To be fulfilled at this level, we need to be able to be our true self. The following tips lay at the identity level and will help you address how you identify with who you are.

TIP #21:
STOP SAYING: "I AM FAT."

21 If saying that we are overweight makes us overweight, then saying that we are thin will make us thin.	True This chapter shows that how we see and identify ourselves impacts our weight.

You get up in the morning, start your morning routine slowly getting out of sleep-mode, brush your teeth, have a shower, start to feel fresh and ready for the day ahead, then, bam! Here it is. The mirror. Reflecting your image at you as you step out of the shower in your Adam and Eve outfit.

You don't recognise the body of the person drying themselves right now. What happened? Where did the young healthy figure go? Then come these thoughts in your head: "I used to be in much better shape, what are these love-handles there for?" and then the most horrible thing happens.

After a while, this image reflected back at you day after day becomes part of who you are. And before you know it, you have developed a new limiting identity. Now, when you get out of the shower and glance at yourself, you think: "I am fat." These three simple words could be said with an inoffensive intention, and yet, you have just read how detrimental they can be.

Associating our own identity with a state that doesn't serve you is never a very good idea.

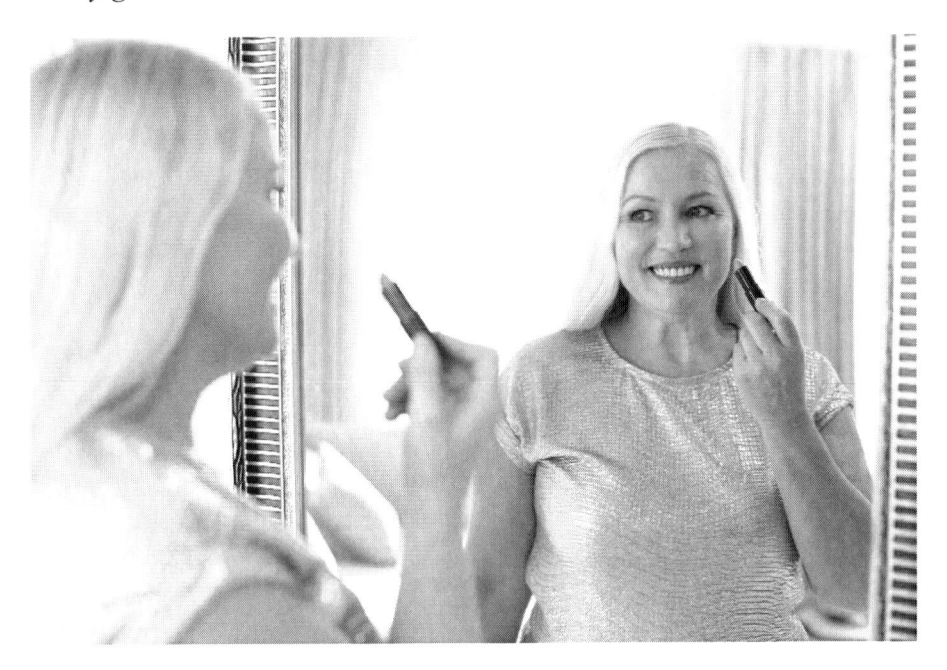

Next time you hear yourself say or think these words, make sure to catch yourself and create an affirmation to counteract its effect.

Rephrase your thoughts. If you happen to hear: "I am fat" in your head, quickly repeat: "This is not my normal. I am in the process of getting back to my normal weight." "I used to let myself go, and now I am on my way to regaining what I once had." "I am determined to get to my ideal weight. "This reflection is temporary. Now, I am on my way to getting back on track."

TIP #22:
LOVE YOURSELF MORE THAN THE FOOD

22 You have to love healthy food.	**False** This statement could be right, in the way that of course, we need to love healthy food. However, this chapter is about loving ourselves, more than we love the food. Enjoy.

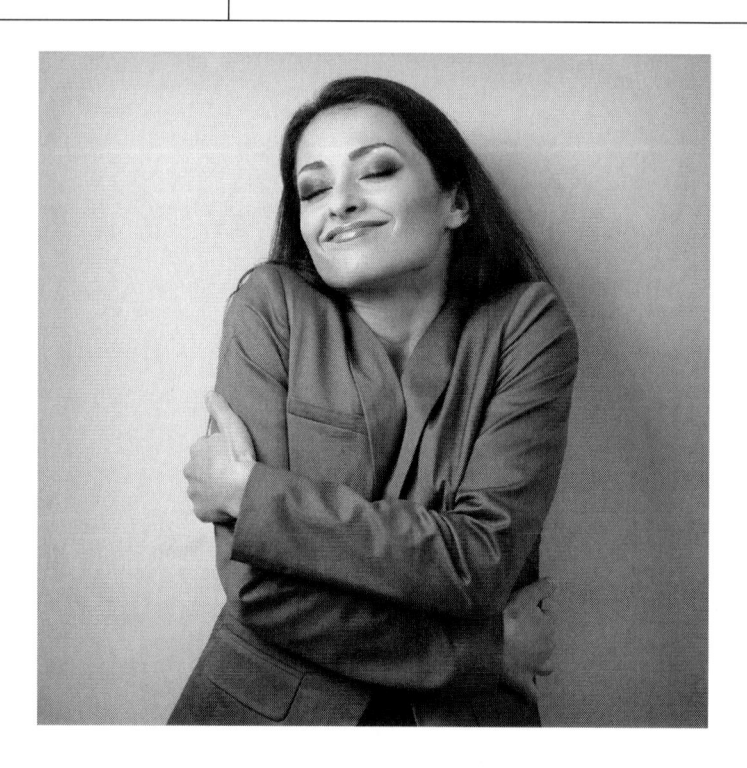

Love who you are. Love being healthy. Love being fit. Love yourself. When you truly love yourself, you can say with confidence: "I love myself a lot more than this piece of cake." Make yourself so important that it becomes a no-brainer when the temptation arises.

Pretend you are driving home after work one night and that there is a tree on the road. Your street is blocked, and there is no way you can keep going. Instead of turning around and saying: "Well, that is too bad, I won't be able to go home. I have to turn around and go back to work I guess. That is sad because I kind of liked my home. And I will never see my kids and family again. I really loved them, but such is life. This tree is keeping me from going back home. I bet it was too good to be true and maybe it was not for me in the first place".

This sounds funny, right? In real life, you would more likely find your way home. You would turn around and find a different route. You would get out of your car and walk if you had to. Or you would find a chainsaw and cut the tree if everything else failed. But you would not give up on your kids and your family as easy as that. The obstacle on the road would not keep you from something so crucial as going home.

Make your goal of being healthy so compelling that it becomes as important to you as your home. YOU are your home. Getting back to YOU has to be so sincere a desire that when an obstacle comes, like the tree on the road, you will take out the chainsaw or do whatever it takes to surmount the barrier.

When you see some food that you should not have, think about how much you love your health. Think of YOU as your home. Keep going when the obstacle shows up. Even if the food is appealing, YOU must be even more attracted to you than to you are to the food.

TIP #23:

BE ALLERGIC

23 Lying is a good thing.	**True** This is only true in a particular context. You will see what I mean about 'lying' in the upcoming chapter.

I sometimes work in elementary schools, teaching kids about self-confidence and respect through movement and music. I love the school environment; the teachers, principals and support staff are all so patient and inspiring. They are forming our future. The work they do with the kids is priceless. I have eternal respect for them and what they do.

I also have one more reason to shake my head and wonder how they do it. I am referring to how they manage to stay healthy with the number of constant temptations presenting themselves in the teachers' lounge. If you are a teacher or if you have been in a teachers' lounge, you will agree that some schools are a calorie paradise. When children bring treats to their teacher, it always ends up on the tables in the teachers' room. Every day, at recess and lunch, these treats look at you and yell your name until you finally give in and grab a bite, like everyone else.

I have developed a strategy. I lie. When I get offered a piece of chocolate, or cake or pie, or homemade Nanaimo bar, etc., I respond: "No thank you, I am allergic." It eliminates a lot of discussions back and forth. Firstly, it prevents me from sounding like the 'food snob' who responds: "No, I don't eat that, it is not healthy".

It would make everyone feel pretty bad as they are finishing their bite. I certainly don't need to be letting them know that they are making a terrible mistake in leaving these treats around all the time. It is none of my business. It is there. I cannot control the environment I am in. However, I can control my reaction to it. And in saying that I'm allergic, it shuts down the conversation. Instead of the response: "Come one, just one bite won't kill you", the 'allergic' word somehow diffuses all come-backs.

Secondly, if by any chance, I spend too much time in the teachers' lounge and suddenly start being tempted to reach out for a piece of chocolate, I am quickly reminded by my inner-voice: "Well, you can't have one now because you just told everyone that you were allergic." The desire to keep my strategy secret and not uncover my lie is stronger than the desire to eat the sweets. It works for me. Try it.

PART 7:

LIFE PURPOSE (The Big Why)

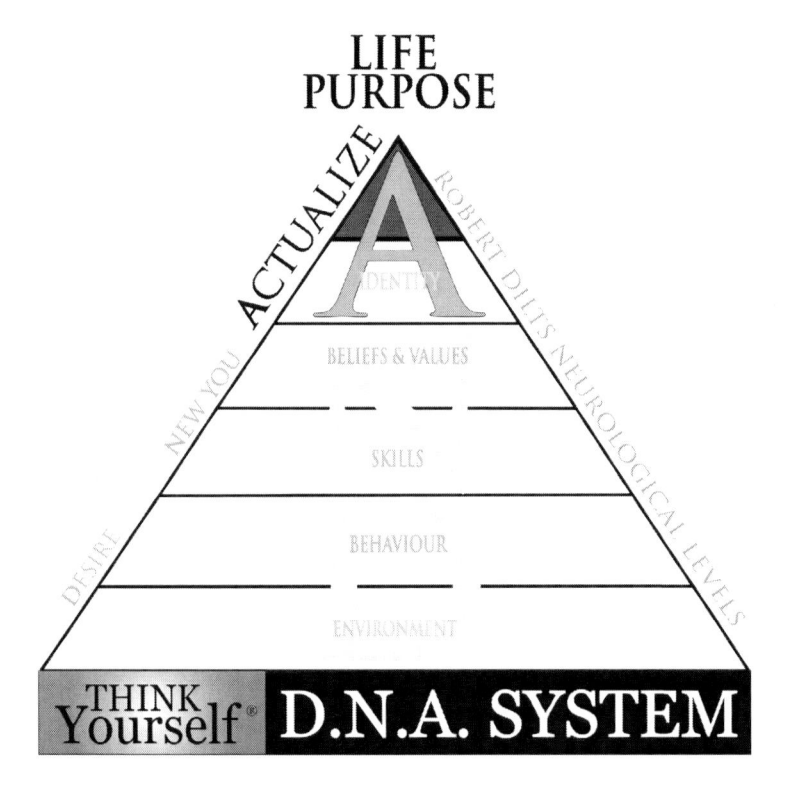

LIFE PURPOSE

Pyramid diagram — Think Yourself® D.N.A. SYSTEM — showing levels from top to bottom: Identity, Beliefs & Values, Skills, Behaviour, Environment. Labeled around the pyramid: ACTUALIZE, NEW YOU, DESIRE, ROBERT DILTS NEUROLOGICAL LEVELS.

When all the layers of the pyramid are aligned, and we live in a wanted environment, doing what we are good at, and following our beliefs and values, then we can feel like we can be ourselves and live our full identity. That is when we can reach our life purpose.

Your life purpose is the reason why you were put on this earth. Who else are you serving? What is beyond yourself? Who else are you serving in your life? What cause is close to your heart?

In Life Purpose, we understand that we are co-creators and co-conspirators in this game called Life. We know why we are here, what we are here to do, who we are here to serve, and we live our life's purpose.

People who are living their 'Why' with a strong sense of conviction inspire confidence, trust and safety. People want to be around people living their purpose because success emanates from a deep place within them. Living our purpose is to live from a place of authenticity.

TIP #24:
KNOW WHY YOU WANT TO BE HEALTHY

24 Focus on what to do to be healthy.	**False** Sorry, I keep doing this to you. This chapter is about focusing on why we want to be healthy instead of focusing on what to do to get there.

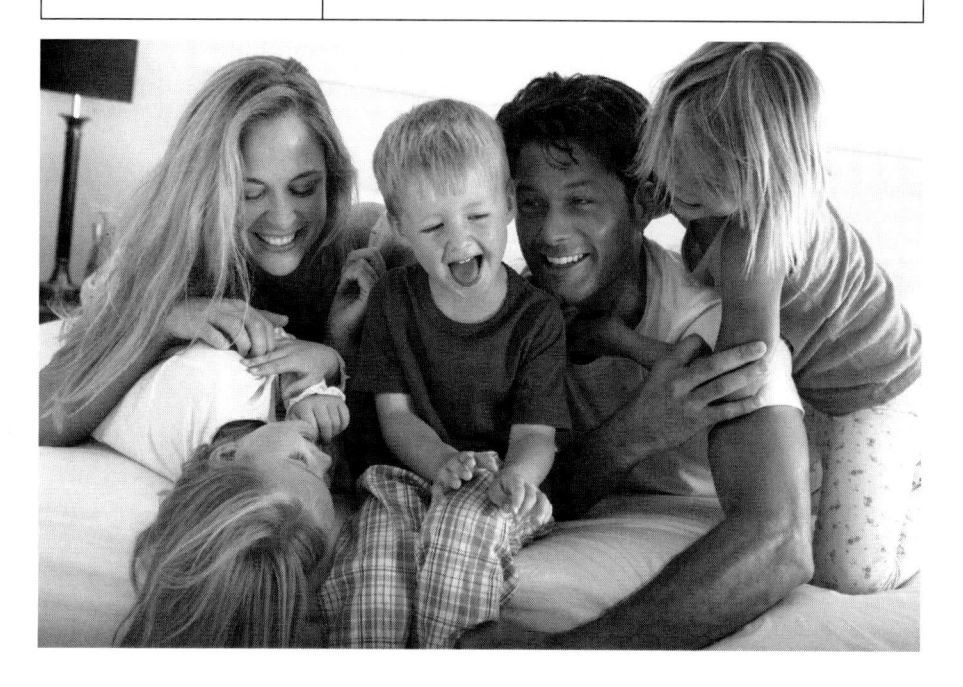

A young child sits in the kitchen, hungry. This kitchen is a sombre place, as the bare cupboards contain the strict minimum and the fridge only has two long sandwiches that his parents and his brothers will be sharing for the rest of the week, until his father gets paid on Friday and can afford to purchase a few groceries. This child's whole childhood is tainted with the memories of food scarcity, and today, as an adult, he does kitchen renovations. He found his life's purpose in making kitchens be a place of fun family times.

Whenever he finishes working in a kitchen, he fills up the refrigerator and the cupboards with groceries, making sure to deliver a full experience where the abundance of food will keep his clients from experiencing the sadness he felt as a kid. He goes to work every day with such a compelling life purpose that the minor obstacles don't even touch the surface of how far he is willing to go to achieve his goal.

What is your big WHY? What are you doing this for? Who do you want to be healthy for? Do you have grandkids that you want to be able to hold? Do you have kids that you want to inspire? Do you want to be a role model for women who are going through something that you overcame yourself? Do you want to reverse the effects of sad experiences in your childhood and inspire young people to keep going if that were to happen to them? Did you witness your parents pass too early and want to make sure you will be there for your kids? What is your story?

Knowing the reason why you want to be healthy is the first step towards making your efforts attractive to you.

TIP #25:
THINK ABOUT THE FUTURE, HOW LONG YOU WANT TO LIVE

25 Thinking about the present will help you get to your ideal weight.	**False** This statement would be correct in many different contexts. What I am addressing here is how thinking about the future will help you get to your ideal weight.

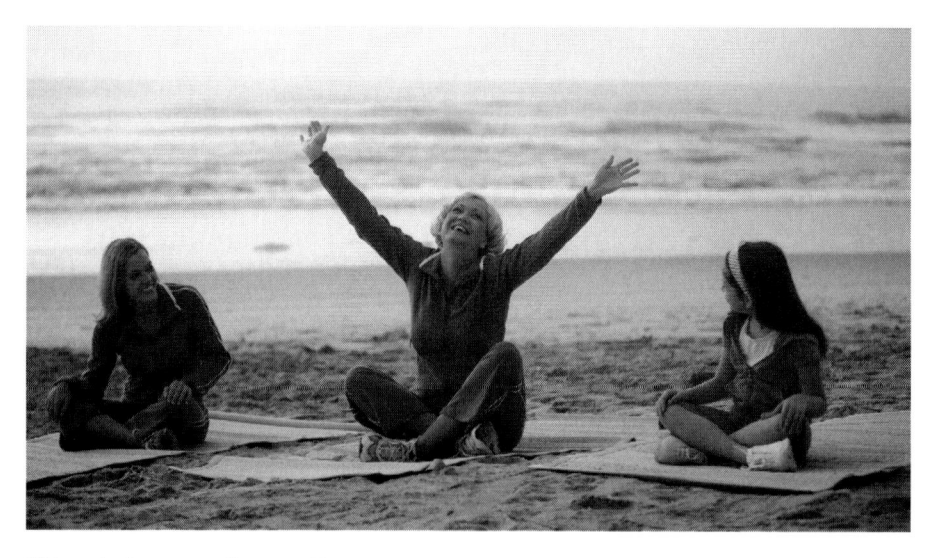

What is in store for you?

When you think about the future, how long do you want to live? How well do you want to age? How free do you want to feel in your eighties, nineties? Do you have parents or grandparents struggling with their health? Do you notice how quality of life can be improved significantly when you are healthy? How many times do you hear older people tell you to take care of your health?

Quality of life as you age is everything. Just the thought of one day having to wear a diaper will help some people make great choices in their forties. Losing our dignity is a prime motivator. I knew a man with a terminal illness who refused treatment just to avoid losing his dignity. He wanted to go on his own terms. He regretted a lot of the poor choices he made while there was still time and yet, he decided to let himself succumb to the illness. If only that dignity power had kicked in a few years earlier, he may have had been able to save himself from such a sad end.

Do you want to be an older person who still lives at home and enjoys your loved ones' company, doing activities together? Do you want to have fewer health concerns? Do you want to have a healthy mind, remember your close ones and the conversations you have with them? Do you want peace of mind, knowing you are not a burden for people around you? Do you want to feel vibrant? Health will energise you and help you keep a positive attitude as you age.

TIP #26:

TEACH OTHERS, BE THE LEADER OF A GROUP, HAVE PEOPLE WHO LOOK UP TO YOU

26 You should think of what other people would think about you.	**True** I always seem to find the one context for a weird statement like this to be true, right? What I am referring to here is how being in a leadership position will give you energy that you may not have thought you had without anyone under your responsibility.

Knowing that other people rely on you adds to the level of commitment you have. When you are serving other people, when other people are counting on you, you find the tenacity you need to get you to the next level.

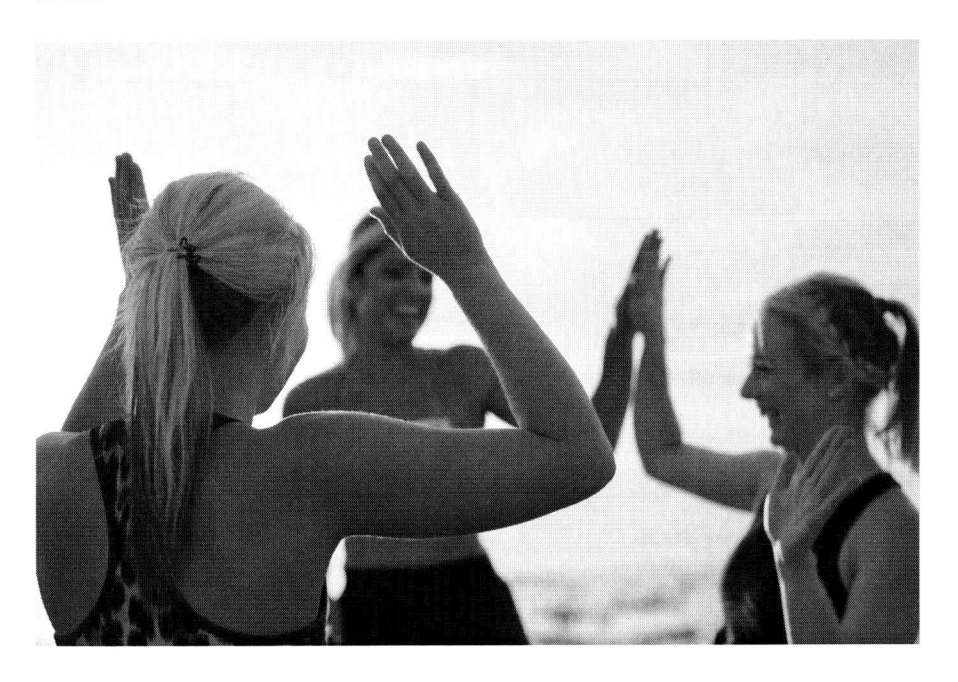

I have been teaching fitness classes for over thirty years. People would say that I like it. Of course I do. Now to say that I do feel like it in every single class and that it never happens that sometimes I would rather stay home, would be a lie. I too have rough days sometimes and would gladly skip. Teaching classes has been my strategy for the past three decades.

Being in that position, where people are counting on me for their workout, makes me want to show up. It is enough to inspire me. All the participants in my classes are showing up week after week, sometimes they miss, but others are there, and they are committed to their health. They want to be there. Unlike me, not only do they show up voluntarily (as they don't have to be there to teach the class) but they also pay for it. They spend money for me to show up and take them through an hour-long fun or strenuous, or both, journey. I cannot let them down. It seriously makes me push myself and show up on my best behaviour.

Doing it for someone else is very powerful. Feeling needed. Feeling like you matter and that without you, someone else could be missing out. Whenever I don't feel like going to my exercise, I tell myself: "I have to show up for them. They need me there more than my need for a break."

I am simply sharing my strategy with you. It doesn't mean that you need to become a fitness instructor. However, you can find a group of friends who want to commit to their health. Put yourself in a leadership position. Be the one that calls the others or invites them for a walk every Tuesday night. As the 'leader' of the group, you have no choice but to show up.

Even when they are not with you and cannot witness, do what they would expect you to be doing. Whenever challenges happen in my life, it is always the thought of those who look up to me that inspires me to keep going.

One year at a fitness expo, I had the chance to see my absolute idol, Lisa Osborne. I was feeling like a kid, or a groupie at a rock concert, cherishing the picture I had been able to take with my hero. I was standing in line to buy a new pair of runners at the expo, when a lady came towards me with excitement and told her girlfriend: "That's her, that's Nathalie, OMG, please take a picture with my fitness instructor, she is so awesome!!!" I turned around and looked behind me to whom this woman was referring. Then I realized it was me.

Surprised, I smiled and let my 'fan' take a picture with me and ironically was thinking how weird it was that somehow, the very same experience I just had with my own idol was replicating itself a few minutes later. I thought: "Tell her, I am really nobody, I am just a fitness instructor…but for this woman, I guess I am more than I thought I was."

I always remember that moment, reminding myself that whatever I do, someone is looking up and I must be my best to meet the expectations of my 'fans' and mainly my own expectations. Who is looking up to you? Who would be proud of you if they saw you right now?

It is when we are not our best that we feel miserable or inadequate. It is not when we make mistakes or when we learn something we don't know. It is the times when we know better and we disappoint ourselves, that we take it hard. I thrive when I know the opportunity to inspire is there. When faced with a decision-making process, I always ask myself the question: "What would someone who needs to be inspired expect me to do here?"

TIP #27:
EAT ORGANIC FOR THE ENVIRONMENT

27 Being healthy will help future generations	False Eating healthy food doesn't only help you live a fantastic free life. It can also be linked to the health of the planet. Here is how.

When talking about life purpose, I can't help but mention the legacy that we leave behind as a user of this beautiful planet Mother Earth.

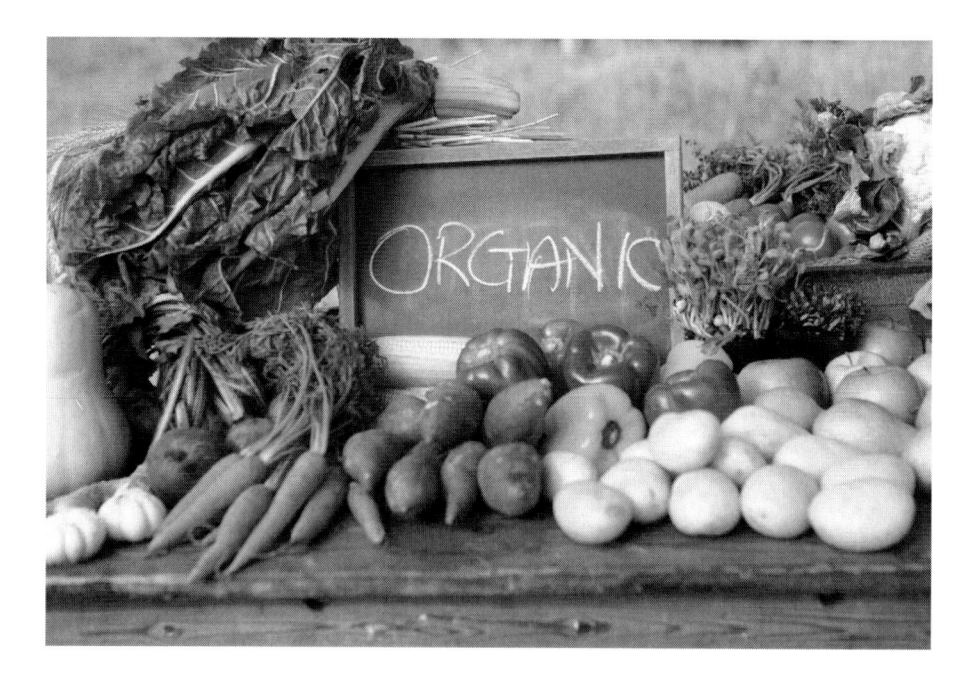

You decide what is important to you. Sometimes, when comparing prices, we get discouraged from the whole 'organic' thing. We feel that we can't afford it or sometimes we feel that it doesn't make sense. There are lots of products out there that are not healthy. Organic or not. An organic bag of chips is still a bag of deep fried potatoes. Stay away from it. Organic doesn't mean healthy. Develop the skills to know the difference.

My husband and I decided a long time ago that it did not matter what kind of car we drove, what kind of house we lived in, or what brand of clothes we wore: what matters to us is what we put in our bodies. Our health is what matters the most. What person, old, rich, and sick, would not give all their fortune for health? At home, we eat organic whenever possible.

Eating organic food goes beyond just thinking about your health. It involves the way the food was grown, how it was harvested, it ensures the sustainability of the way it was produced and the protection of our environment.

As a start, you can try to get your produce organic. Some produce is more likely to be sprayed with pesticides, so you should try to buy them organic. If you can't afford to buy all your fruit organic, see the list below of the twenty fruit and veggies with the most pesticides.

Regardless, wash your food, even if it's organic. It has touched other things in the store, in your car, on the delivery truck, and it was touched by other people too.

The 20 fruits and veggies with the most pesticides

Some produce you should always buy organic to avoid pesticides. Ranked in order by the Environmental Working Group (EWG) with the worst at the top are peaches.

1. Peaches
2. Apples
3. Sweet bell peppers
4. Celery
5. Nectarines
6. Strawberries
7. Cherries
8. Pears
9. Grapes (imported)
10. Spinach
11. Lettuce
12. Potatoes
13. Carrots
14. Green beans
15. Hot peppers
16. Cucumbers
17. Raspberries
18. Plums
19. Grapes (domestic)
20. Oranges

The 20 fruits and veggies with the least pesticides

According to EWG, the following fruits and vegetables have the lowest pesticide load, ranked in order with the one with the absolute lowest pesticides first.

1. Onion
2. Avocado
3. Sweet corn (frozen)
4. Pineapples
5. Mango
6. Asparagus
7. Sweet peas (frozen)
8. Kiwi
9. Bananas
10. Cabbage
11. Broccoli
12. Papaya
13. Blueberries
14. Cauliflower
15. Winter squash
16. Watermelon
17. Sweet potatoes
18. Tomatoes
19. Honeydew melon
20. Cantaloupe

SOME FINAL TIPS

- Eat often–every two to three hours (complex carbs and lean proteins) and drink water.

- Fibre and fat (essential fatty acids) are your best buddies.

- Eat at home. Keep a full fridge or use a cooler to go.

- Prepare, prepare, prepare!

- Use smaller plates to help control portion sizes (9-inch plates).

- Never skip breakfast and never starve.

- Exercise four to five times a week (with others whenever possible).

- Set up short-term goals and tell the whole world! It will help you commit to your plan. Tell people you don't eat bad food–at work, at home, or socially.

- Avoid refined, processed, and sugar-loaded foods.

- Eat real food! Complement with vitamins and supplements.

MY MEALS

As people always ask me exactly what I eat, I thought I would include this as a bonus chapter for you.

MY BREAKFAST

This book is not intended as a recipe book. Far from it. However, I still get lots of emails and questions about what I eat, specifically. The next few chapters will give you tips on what I eat on a regular basis. You will be amazed at the lack of variety. I am so accustomed to my meals that I simply repeat them over and over and just love it. When I go away, I crave them and can't wait to get home to be back to make my own salad. I also included a chapter, later on, about what I order in a restaurant.

Here are my favourite breakfast options:

Oatmeal

As mentioned in chapter one, I make steel-cut oatmeal in advance and have it ready to go in the fridge. I simply have to put a dollop of it in a saucepan and add a bit of soy milk, berries and half a banana.

Avoid adding sugar. It may take you a while to get used to the taste of oatmeal without a pound of brown sugar in it. In the transition, you may choose to add a teaspoon of honey or maple syrup or a few dried fruits like cranberries, raisins or dates which will give you sweet yet naturally-occurring sugar in the fruit.

The soy milk (make sure you buy organic) has 6 grams of protein. Even though I know that almond milk and other varieties are really popular, as I don't eat meat, I am seeking for proteins, and there are none or just a little in these beverages. There is a new coconut milk now that has added protein in it. That would be a perfect option as soon as I can get my hands on it.

I get healthy fibres from the oats, that will be used as a filter for everything else I will be eating for the remainder of the day. I get healthy fats and proteins from sprouted chia and hemp hearts I added when I cooked the oats.

Shake

A few days a week, I eat a shake for breakfast. I make my own protein powder with a mix of the following: pea protein powder, rice protein powder, Acai powder, Red Maca powder, Spirulina & Chlorella powder, wheatgrass powder and hemp hearts. I mix all the powders and keep the mix in a glass container in the fridge. I scoop it into my Vitamix in the morning with frozen berries and half a banana, kale or any greens or fruit I have in the fridge. This breakfast option allows me to either eat on the go or bring my breakfast to my office as I can sip it while I work. My days usually start at 5 a.m. as I have early clients from eastern time zones for whom it is already time for their coaching session.

I also use the same powder mix just with water for my pre-workout fuel or between two classes.

Cereals

I also like a bowl of cereal once in a while, although it is hard to find cereals without sugar. You may have to try a few before you get used to one that you enjoy. Remember, this old habit of eating sweet things in the morning needs to go.

I like Ezekiel cereals, puffed quinoa, puffed rice, Whole "O"s, and Smart Bran with psyllium cereal by Nature's Path.

Again, I use soy milk and half a banana or berries to sweeten the flavour and add a fruit serving.

Scrambled eggs

Sometimes, on the weekend, my husband makes us an omelette or scrambled eggs. He mixes whatever vegetables we have: spinach, broccoli, peppers, mushrooms or onion, and water-fries them in a pan first, then adds the scrambled eggs. Egg-white is a mistake. Use the whole egg. The yolk contains the perfect amount of fat to digest the protein included in the egg white. If you are concerned about your cholesterol, lower your animal protein intake from meat. The eggs are inoffensive.

MY LUNCH

I eat the very same salad every day. I love it. It consists of arugula, spinach, half an avocado, a scoop of cooked quinoa, half a cup of beets, a hard-boiled egg, and one tbsp each of chopped walnut, basil-olive oil, maple syrup, and lemon juice.

Sometimes, I add goat feta cheese when I feel like celebrating, corn when in season, chickpeas when I am out of quinoa or eggs, or mango when in season.

In the winter, I sometimes make my salad smaller and eat soup with it. I would make a big pot of soup on the weekend with all the veggies I can get my hands on, that I add to previously-cooked beans (lima beans or chickpeas, washed twice, then cooked in my slow cooker with onions while I work all day).

OTHER LUNCH IDEAS

- Acorn squash or butternut squash soup (simply steam and puree in blender), add Belsoy dairy-free cream and fresh basil.

- A gluten-free wrap with chickpeas, sprouts, spinach, avocado, tomato, plain Greek yoghurt.

- Grilled organic chicken breasts, cut into cubes and stored in individual portions. My husband uses these to add meat to any of my vegetarian choices.

MY SNACKS

- Apples. I am hooked on Pink Ladies. To me, now that I have experienced the sweet and sour perfect combo of a Pink Lady, there is no going back to any other apples. I eat one every day. I love them!

- A quarter of an avocado with crackers (choose rice cake, Ryvita or crackers with low sodium and no sugar).

- Veggie sticks ready in the fridge – if I feel like a big snack, with a pureed avocado or pureed chickpeas.

- Hard boiled eggs on crackers.

- Half an avocado with Raincoast tuna, mixed with plain Greek yoghurt (instead of mayo) in the pit-hole.

- Medjool dates.

- Almonds, pecans, walnuts, pistachios, macadamia nuts.

PRE/POST-WORKOUT SHAKES.

The same protein power as in the breakfast above except that I only mix it with water and put only one scoop. I drink a shake before exercising, especially in the morning and in-between workouts when I teach two classes back-to-back. See the powder mix, from the breakfast section above, mixed with water.

MY DINNER

I eat the same salad as my lunch salad above. Soup. And sometimes vegetable stir-fries or roasted vegetables.

As you can see, my meals are very repetitive, and I like it this way. By knowing the taste of what you eat, you eat less of it. It is when presented with a new food that you tend to overeat.

Other dinner options I cook once in a while.

- Chickpeas (put in a slow cooker in the morning with water and onion, so they are ready for dinner) with butternut squash and yams in cubes, curry powder.

- Brown rice or quinoa. Pop into a rice cooker with the vegetables in the veggie steamer on top to be ready when you get back from a fitness class, and by the time you get out of the shower, the rice and the veggies are ready.

- Veggie burgers (quinoa, shredded carrots, zucchini, mushrooms, egg) with Portobello mushroom as a bun.

- Lentils, lima beans, split pea stews with veggies (again, slow cooked).

- Spaghetti squash cut in half with mushrooms in the hole, served with homemade quinoa spaghetti sauce. (I also use quinoa to make meat-loaves or sometimes I mix the quinoa with half of the organic extra-lean ground beef if I have meat-eaters coming over.)

- A beautiful piece of wild fish grilled with salad and veggies. However, I tend to eat less and less of fish as the sourcing becomes more and more debatable.

- Homemade pizza on pita bread with ricotta cheese, chicken (on one half for my husband), shredded carrots, onion, mushrooms, bocconcini cheese or goat cheese, tomatoes and peppers on top.

- Zucchini-pasta with quinoa-meatball tomato sauce.

DESSERTS

- Date

- Fruit (mango is my favourite).

- Greek yoghurt with fruit.

- Raspberry pie (crust made with cereal in the blender and coconut oil, and fresh raspberries, plain Greek yoghurt on top sweetened with maple syrup).

- Date squares made without sugar. Organic oats, gluten-free flour and coconut oil (or butter) for the top and bottom. Pitted dates pureed with pure blueberry juice for the middle. Cook in the oven for 30 to 40 minutes or until golden.

- Oatmeal and dates cookies made without sugar. Coconut oil, egg, soy milk, gluten-Free flour, soda, cinnamon, oats, chopped dates. If the kids come over or we have company, I add a mashed banana to make them a bit sweeter.

NATHALIE PLAMONDON-THOMAS

"You are AWESOME! End Negative Self-Talk & Live to Your Full Potential!" www.thinkyourself.com

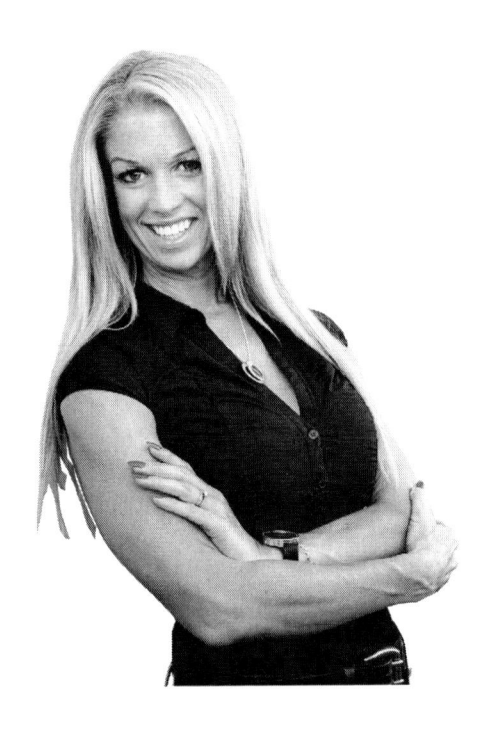

We know exactly what to do, and yet, do the reverse. Nathalie is the Expert with a Proven System to reprogram your brain and get you transformational results.

Founder of the THINK Yourself® ACADEMY, Speaker, Publisher, Master Life Coach and No.1 International Best-Selling Author of 15 books on wellness and empowerment, Nathalie combines 10 years of experience in human resources, 25 years in sales and 30 years in the fitness industry. In 2007, she was "Fitness Instructor of the Year" for Canada. She uses neuroscience in her practice as a Master Life Coach, Executive Coach and Transformation Coach to reprogram your brain to end self-sabotage and live to your full potential.

"You can take a horse to water, but you can't make him drink".

Somehow, Nathalie can.

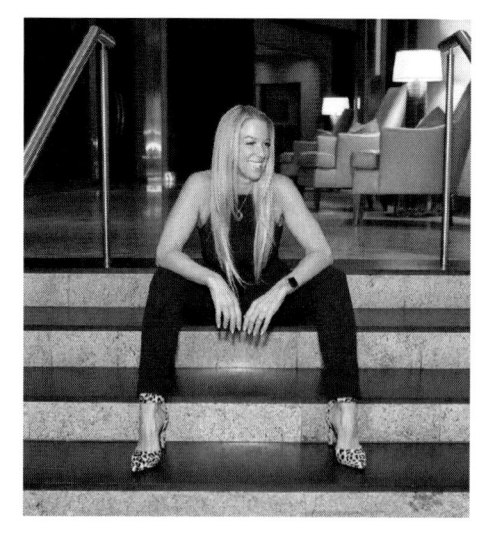

"Hi, I'm Nathalie.

My parents were freaks!!!

They never put a gate by the stairs when my brother and I were babies because they never wanted to imply that we could fall. They didn't say: "Don't fall"; They would say: "Be careful around there." If they needed me to bring a full glass of water to the table they would just say: "Use a strong firm hand and bring this glass to the table," instead of creating anxiety around the action of carrying the water by saying: "Don't spill it!"

There were signs everywhere in the house with motivational phrases like: "You can be everything you want"; "Yes you can"; "You will miss 100% of the shots you won't take"; "If you're going to do it, do it right", etc.

On Sundays, we didn't go to church (although we are Christian Catholics). Instead, my parents would make us sit in the living room to listen to motivational tape cassettes from Jean-Marc Chaput, Zig Ziglar, Og Mandino, etc. Needless to say, I was brainwashed into positive thinking at a very young age.

I believe that my life purpose is to motivate, inspire and support people to discover that they have everything inside themselves in order to be their best and live to their full potential.

I got my first 'calling' to help people at a very young age. My parents would not read us Disney stories at night. They would either sing us a song to put us to sleep with their guitar (which explains my love for music), or they would tell us motivational stories. Here is my favourite bedtime story: It is about an old man on the beach, who was throwing starfish back into the sea, one by one. A little girl asked him: "What are you doing sir?" and the old man responded: "I am saving the starfish from dying, as the tide brought them to shore, they will dry and die if I don't throw them back in the sea."

The little girl looked at the endlessly long beach and said: "But sir, no offence, but there are so many, you can't save them all! It doesn't really make a difference."

The old man responded, as he was showing the little girl the starfish that he was holding in his hands: "Well my dear, for this particular starfish, it makes a whole world of difference."

I was thinking: "When I grow up, I will be a starfish saviour and save them all, one at a time!" And the rest is history.

I was born in Saint-Raymond, a small town near Quebec City, Canada. I lived in Quebec for a big chunk of my life as a successful entrepreneur in the printing industry, with over 50 employees, mastering human resources and sales techniques until I moved to Toronto, Ontario in my twenties, where I got seriously into fitness, personal training and nutrition consultation all while accumulating 16 more years of experience in sales in the natural food industry.

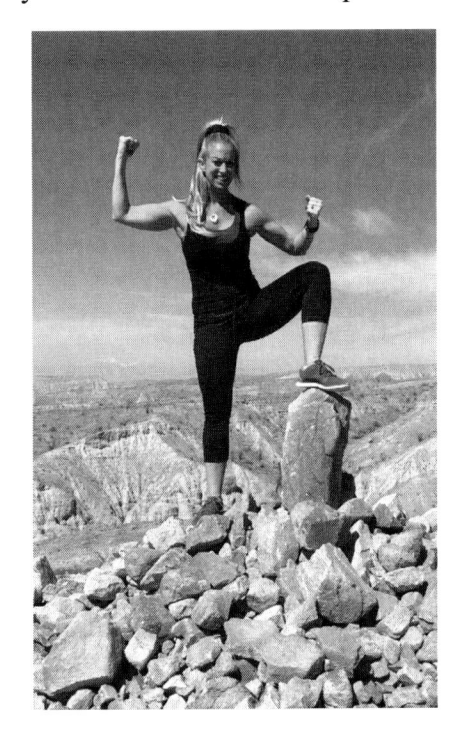

After reaching the top of my game as the No.1 Fitness Instructor in Canada, I realized that being my own personal best wasn't fulfilling me. I started to realize that even though I was helping people, my clients were not successful because I was giving them a better kale salad recipe or showing them a different way of doing push-ups. They thrived because they were changing the way they thought. Their mindset was influenced by mine.

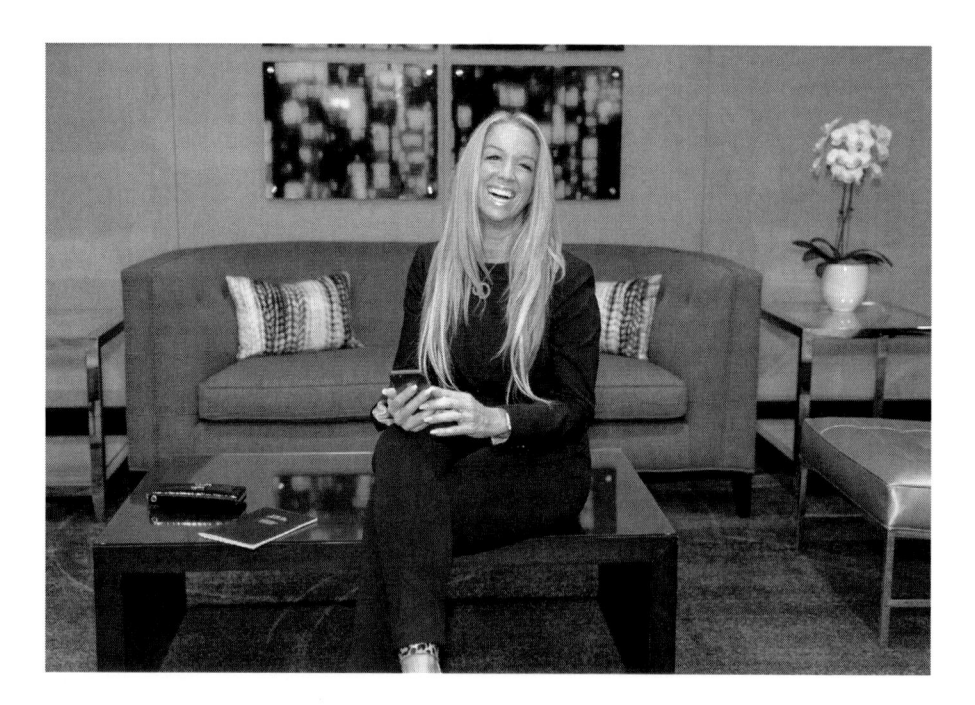

I then started to study neuroscience and the astonishing powers of the brain. I got a Neuro-Linguistic Programming (NLP) Master certification and Life Coaching certifications and have spent the last 10 years developing a system combining my experience as an entrepreneur, my health and wellness knowledge and the specific processes I use with the thousands of clients I have helped to reach their full potential.

I work with clients one-on-one and propel people into the life they want through my coaching, books, events and speaking engagements. I also continue to teach fitness classes, 30 years and counting, using fitness as an introductory platform in order to help people be their best.

Ten years ago, I also started to work with kids in schools, which gives me even more opportunity to impact and improve people's lives, as I believe if certain values are planted at a young age, flourishing happens sooner in life.

I also co-authored a ready-to-use learning resource to build self-esteem and perseverance. "THINK Yourself® POSITIVE – The Adventures of Captain Vic" is dedicated to teachers from Kindergarten to Grade four and parents of children between 5 and 10 years old. I am convinced that by transforming children's inner language, they will increase their potential for success in life.

I now live in White Rock, British Columbia with my loving husband Duff and we are celebrating our 18th anniversary this year."

NATHALIE P.

nathalie@thinkyourself.com
www.thinkyourself.com
https://www.facebook.com/nathalie.plamondonthomas
https://www.facebook.com /ThinkYourselfAcademy/
https://www.linkedin.com/in/nathalie-plamondon-thomas-6b3262a/
instagram: @nathaliepthinkyourself
twitter: @thinkyourselfac

THINK Yourself® ACADEMY

NATHALIE PLAMONDON-THOMAS

Transformation Expert

8 times International Bestselling Author

nathalie@thinkyourself.com

www.thinkyourself.com

https://www.facebook.com/nathalie.plamondonthomas

https://www.facebook.com /ThinkYourselfAcademy/

https://www.linkedin.com/in/nathalie-plamondon-thomas-6b3262a/

instagram: @nathaliepthinkyourself

twitter: @thinkyourselfac

Book your FREE 15-min Virtual Coffee:
www.thinkyourself.com/schedule

You can find more from the THINK Yourself® series on
www.thinkyourself.com:

THINK Yourself® SUCCESSFUL

THINK Yourself® THIN

THINK Yourself® CLEAN from the Inside Out

THINK Yourself® GRATEFUL

THINK Yourself® HEALTHY

THINK Yourself® POSITIVE for KIDS (for parents)

THINK Yourself® POSITIVE for KIDS (for teachers)

FROM THE SAME AUTHOR

THINK Yourself® THIN

THINK Yourself® SUCCESSFUL

THINK Yourself® GRATEFUL

THINK Yourself® HEALTHY

THINK Yourself® CLEAN from the Inside Out

THINK Yourself® A RELATIONSHIPS PRO

EN SANTÉ PAR LA PENSÉE

SHINE

SIMPLE SUCCESS STRATEGIES

WHEN YOU'RE HUNGRY, YOU GOTTA EAT

QUAND ON A FAIM, IL FAUT MANGER

Children's Resources:

THINK Yourself® POSITIVE
The Adventures of Captain Vic – for Teachers

THINK Yourself® POSITIVE
The Adventures of Captain Vic – for Parents

POSITIF PAR LA PENSÉE
Les Aventures de Capitaine Vic – pour enseignants

POSITIF PAR LA PENSÉE
Les Aventures de Capitaine Vic – pour parents

THANK YOU

Thank you to my clients, for allowing me to be part of your journey, trusting me and causing me to grow as we walk together towards our life purpose. You keep me honest and on point.
I am forever grateful to you.

Thank you to my parents Micheline and Yves Plamondon for your constant inspiration and support, and for being at the head of my 'fan-club'. You are always there for me and bring me so much energy.

Finally, thank you to my husband Duff Thomas for your continuous support and unconditional love. Once in a lifetime, you meet someone you want to share your soul with and despite them knowing everything about you, they love you anyways. Thank you, Duff. I love you too!

Nathalie